The Patient's Guide to Dental Implants

Why to Choose Dental Implants, What is the Process, and How to Care for Them

By Katrina M. Schroeder, D.M.D

Copyright page

Dedication

To Charles Schroeder, for allowing me to use him as my example patient for so many things, supporting me through college, dental school, and in my career, and for being the best dad ever.

Table of contents page

1. Why this guide?
2. Why would I get an implant
3. How to use this guidebook
4. Single tooth implants
5. A few missing teeth
6. Whole Jaw replacement
7. Other considerations
8. Conclusion
9. Dental Implant Dictionary
10. Acknowledgements

The Patient's Guide to Dental Implants

Why to Choose Dental Implants, What is the Process, and How to Care for Them

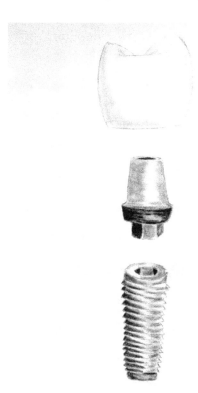

Why this guide?

So you are interested in dental implants. You have probably already looked into some things that are out there, looking online, asking friends and family. A quick google search will bring up a hundred or more websites of dental offices that say something like "yep, we do implants" and everything else is written for dentists with tons of technical terms. What is an abutment? Wait, so the implant is not the whole thing and there are different parts?

And asking friends and family is not much help either. First, not everyone has heard of dental implants. Second, the most common response is that they are expensive. The third is that people worry about having something foreign in their mouth.

But what about the alternatives? Bridges require you to have your other teeth ground down to nubs so that they can have the bridge go over them and they are difficult to keep clean. Dentures and partials, being removable, have to be able to move, so your bite is not stable, and they can come loose at inconvenient times. Plus, dentures and partials cover your gums and roof of mouth, which takes getting used to and lessens the taste of food. None of these are that great sounding either.

So, what do you do? How do you choose? You want to know more about your options but do not know where to start. It is frustrating. Do you go with the old fashioned options, like a denture, and give in to having teeth that you sit in a cup at night like so many sitcom grandmothers? Do you have perfectly good teeth ground down just to replace a few others, or even just to replace one?

I know all of this because I see patients every day that would benefit tremendously from dental implants, but they do not know enough about them to make the decision to improve their dental health. I have helped them research dental implants so that they can see what the parts and processes are. I have researched myself for a good reference for patients to be able to show them, or give them something that they can take with them to show their family. Everything that I have found is either too technical and written for a dentist, or overly simple and not really informative.

So I decided to write book, something written for patients, not for dentists. I want you to know what your options are and why dental implants can be the best of those options. I want you to know what dental implants are, what the process for them is, and how to take care of them afterward. I also want you to know why you would want dental implants over the alternatives. I want all of this for you so that you can make the best decisions about your own dental health.

If you want to be able to make your own best decisions about replacing your teeth, then keep reading.

Why would I get a dental implant?

Dental implants are the closest that you can get to having your natural teeth back. That, in and of itself, is the main reason to have implants to replace your teeth. But what does that really mean? What do teeth do that other restorations don't? Why would I want to replace a tooth in the back that I can't see?

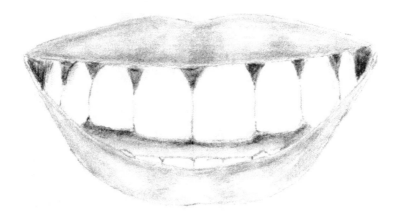

Let us start with what teeth do. There are three things that your teeth provide you: aesthetics, speaking, and eating. Every tooth participates in eating and speaking. For many people, even your first molars can be seen when you smile and laugh, so even back teeth participate in aesthetics.

Aesthetics is how you look, how you smile, how you laugh. It is more than just that, it is confidence with how you look; confidence that your teeth are not going to fall out like a partial or complete denture does or having a gap under a tooth for a bridge. What would it be like for you to never show your teeth when you smile because you are missing one? What would it be like for you to fear that your teeth will fall out when you sneeze or move when you speak? Or what would it be like to have something that replaces your teeth that is part of you,

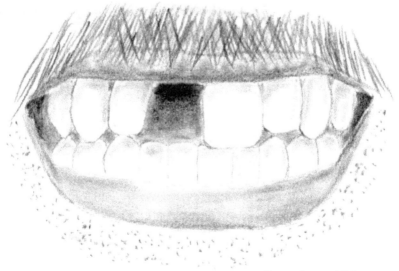

just as your tooth was? What would you prefer, a beautiful, complete smile, or one missing a tooth? Dental implants provide you with a smile, one that you can smile and laugh with confidence and looking just as natural as your own teeth.

Speaking is another issue. This is tooth position. Have you heard a child that has lost their baby tooth whistle while they talk, or sing about wanting their two front teeth for Christmas? Even missing a back tooth makes speech become slushy because your tongue goes into

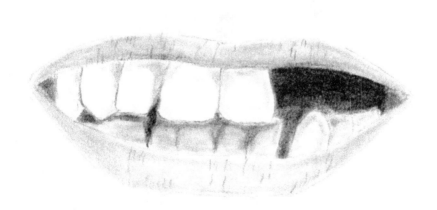

that space. Bridges can help with this and provide a surface for your tongue to find, but they have other detriments that I will review with you shortly. Then there are dentures and partials, if you are missing multiple teeth or all your teeth. Dentures and partials do aid with speech, but they are thick and bulky. They cover parts or the entire roof of your mouth and have flanges on the sides that go down between your gums and cheek or between your gums and tongue. They take up space, which your tongue will have to learn to speak around. Learning to speak with a denture or partial can take months for you to feel that you are speaking normally again. And when the partial or denture wears down and is replaced, you get to learn a new denture all over again.

That leaves eating. Even missing one tooth decreases your ability to chew, and the more teeth that you are missing, the worse it gets. Chewing releases flavor from your food. So how well your food tastes is dependent upon how well you can chew it. Yes, bridges can replace the function for chewing, but not as well as an implant because you can get food stuck under the bridge which can be uncomfortable. Dentures and partials, while they give you a surface to chew with, do not allow you the biting forces that you used to have with teeth. When all of your teeth are removed, the strength that you have to chew with is only one quarter of what it is with teeth. Dentures and partials rest on your gums, and your gums can only take so much pressure. Chewing also affects how much nutrition you get out of your food. When you are missing teeth, even just one, you do not chew your food as well and wind up swallowing larger chunks of food or eating softer foods. Larger chunks of food are harder to digest, while softer foods tend to be more fatty and sugary with fewer nutrients to start with. Remember, missing one molar takes out one quarter of your main chewing teeth.

Yes, there are other options that I have mentioned to replace teeth. These are bridges, if you have a tooth on either side of the missing area, or dentures and partials.

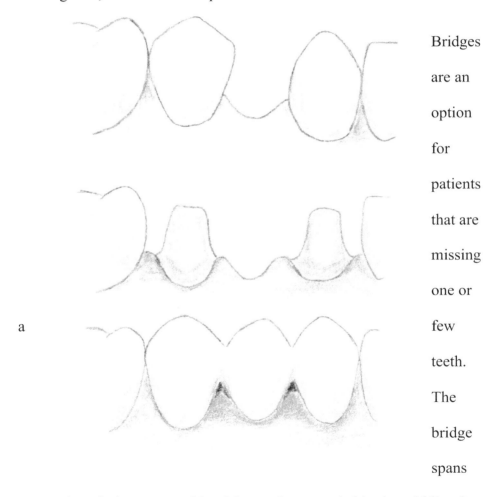

Bridges are an option for patients that are missing a one or few teeth. The bridge spans across the missing space with a fake tooth suspended in the middle of two other teeth. Bridges require your adjacent teeth to be ground down to peg shapes so that the bridge can be cemented over it. This often means grinding down two perfectly good teeth, just to suspend the fake tooth between them. Then there are the other considerations. The ADA has shown that bridges have the shortest average life span of any restoration on natural teeth. This is because bridges are notoriously hard to clean. Food gets under the bridge, bacteria eat the food, and cause cavities and periodontal disease. Then, if something happens to just one of the teeth that is supporting the bridge, you have to replace the whole thing.

Partials and dentures are removable restorations that replace missing teeth. The key here is removable. Because these are removable, they have to be able to move. So the partials and dentures are not as stable as teeth or implants. They move. They also reduce your chewing force, so harder foods are more difficult to chew through. And they cover over the roof of your mouth and your gums. You cannot feel the texture of your food as well. Your ability to taste is reduced. This makes your food less enjoyable. The parts that cover over your gums and the roof of your mouth also take up space so speaking is more difficult and they feel bulky under your lips and along your cheeks.

There is something else, something that you do not see because it happens slowly over time: bone loss. The bone that holds your teeth is there to hold your teeth and the forces of chewing and speaking with your teeth stimulate the bone to stay there. When a tooth is lost, that stimulation of your bone is lost too. Your body then takes your jaw bone away to be put to better use elsewhere. This is why people who have had dentures for a while look so much older, their jaw is deteriorating. This happens even with just one tooth missing. The bone in that area will slowly become indented compared to the adjacent teeth, which lets food collect in that spot. Dentures, partials, and bridges do not fix this. In fact, dentures and partials actually make it go faster than not replacing the teeth at all. Dental implants stimulate your bone just as your teeth do, so they are the only option to replace teeth that also helps to maintain your bone.

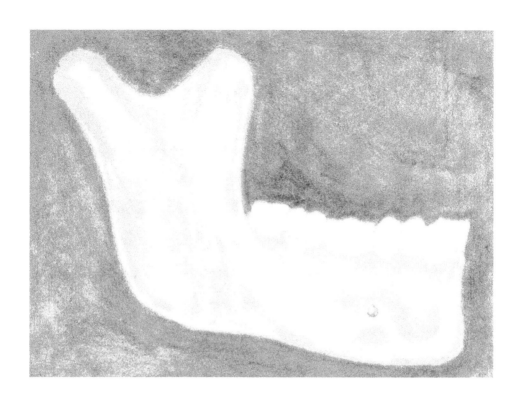

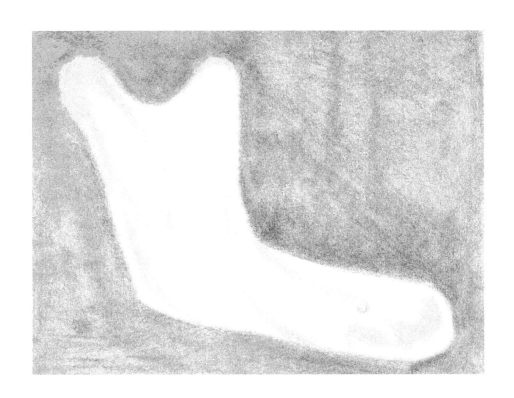

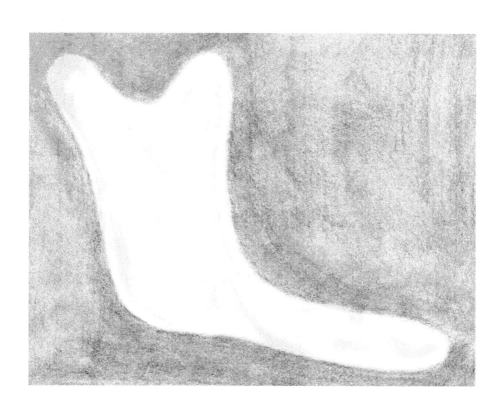

How to use this guide book

Still interested in how to replace your teeth as in a way close to nature as possible? Great! You have found a great resource of information right here. This book is how I review dental implants with my own patients, translating all of the technical terms into regular language. I have also included many of the quick sketches that I have found myself drawing over and over again, just drawn out with more detail for you.

This book is divided into three main sections, one for each of the most common dental implant restoration types: single missing tooth, a few missing teeth, and whole jaw reconstruction. At the end, I do mention some of the other uses for dental implants, some of the new dental implant technologies that are coming and a note on who would not benefit from dental implants.

To use this book, go to the section that applies to you the most. I will repeat myself in each section on some of the aspects of dental implants that pertain to all implants, like osseointegration, so you do not need to jump between sections. I will also translate dental technical terms into regular language so that you will know that osseointegration is the process of your bone and your implant fusing together so that the implant becomes part of you.

Dental implants are the best way to replace missing teeth for most people. They have some of the longest average lifespans of any dental restoration, and with adequate care and maintenance, can last as long as you do.

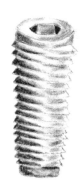

Why have a dental implant?

Dental implants are the closest you can get to having your own natural tooth or teeth back. They are placed into the space where your missing tooth was. The implant replaces the root of your tooth, the part that goes into your bone, and a crown replaces the part of the tooth that you see, just like a crown on a natural tooth. There is a piece, called an abutment, which is a connector between the implant and the crown.

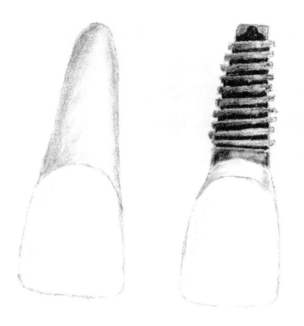

From your standpoint, the dental implant functions just as your tooth did for eating, speaking, and aesthetics. Implants are also some of the longest lasting dental restorations. They are intended to last as long as you do, so they are intended to last for life.

Now, there are other ways of replacing a missing tooth or missing teeth. You could have a removable partial or complete denture. If you are already missing a tooth, then you may already have one of these. These removable replacements, being removable, have to be able to move, so they are never as stable as your own teeth. To keep these stable, they have to cover your gums and may have hooks that hold onto other teeth. And, because they move, it is possible for food to get caught under the denture.

If you are missing some of your teeth, then a bridge, or fixed partial denture, may be an option for replacement for you. First, for most bridges, you have to have at least one tooth on each side of the area you are missing teeth from. Bridges require grinding down these neighboring teeth to attach the bridge across the gap. Bridges also have one of the shortest average life spans in all of dentistry, mostly because they are difficult to clean. Food and bacteria can get under the bridge. If this is not cleaned out, then the bacteria breed and result in cavities and periodontal disease. To clean under the bridge, you will need some special equipment, such as floss threaders or a water irrigation system, and definitely more time than just regular brushing and flossing.

You can avoid all of these issues with dental implants.

Single tooth implants

The single tooth dental implant is the most basic of the tooth replacement options, but that does not make it simple. There is actually a lot of science and planning behind these that allow them to work. I will give you an overview of this a little further ahead.

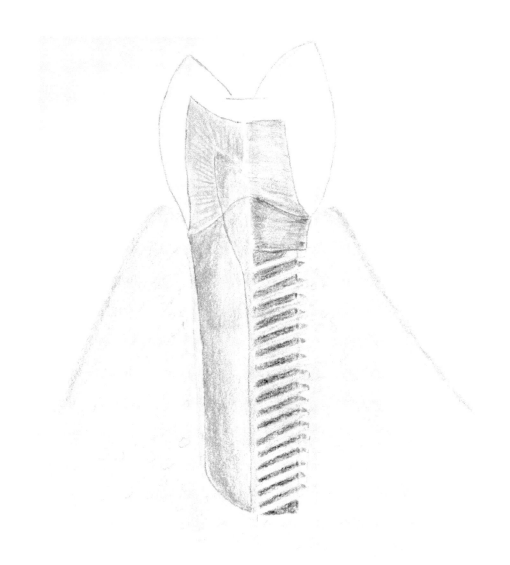

Single tooth dental implants replace a single missing tooth. The implant itself replaces the root of your tooth, the part that goes into your bone. A connector, called an abutment, attaches to the implant and comes up through your gums. A crown, just like a crown on a natural tooth, goes on to the abutment.

The single tooth implant is the closest you can get to having your natural tooth back.

Implant placement consultation and examination

Of course, for an implant to be placed, you either need to be missing a tooth or soon will be missing a tooth if you need a tooth removed. If you are already missing a tooth, that is great. Some of your healing has already started. If you have a tooth that needs to be removed, then that is done first. The specifics of your implant procedures will be discussed with your dentist or surgeon at your consultation, so what I have written here is the usual proceedings.

Yes, you will need an exam of the area before the actual implant placement. This exam will include both visual examination of the area and some form of x-ray. Often, a CT scan of the area is done so that a computer generated three dimensional model of your bone can be viewed and measured. This will be used to determine the size and positioning of your implant as well as if you bone needs any shaping for your best results. Bone shaping can include reshaping your current bone, or grafting on bone if you need more. The visual exam looks for other factors, such as the health of your gums in the area, how visible the implant will be when you smile, the size and shape of your other teeth. You see, dental implants are actually planned and placed based upon how to have as natural an end result as possible for both aesthetics and function.

After your exam, then all the specific factors of your case will be reviewed with you, including if your bone and gums need to be reshaped, if you will need any kind of grafting to add bone or gum tissue, and what your time frame options are. There are certain minimum time frames for healing, but after those minimum times, you usually have some wiggle room.

Please note that I will make reference to your dentist or surgeon. Often dental implants are completed by a team of doctors, one for the surgical components and one for the restorations. This may be in one office or in two. Sometimes, a single doctor will do the whole procedure or you may go to a dental implant center where multiple doctors work together in one office. All of these options can have excellent results. Personally, I do not put in dental implants in my office, however the oral surgeon that I work with is only half a mile from my office and I often go to his office for my patients.

While there are specifics that will be unique to you, there are many things that are the same across all implants, so I will review what the usual circumstances are and note variations where they may come up.

Implant placement

First, you are either already missing a tooth or you will have a tooth removed in the near future. If you are already missing a tooth, then a small incision is made so that your gums can be moved out of the way and your dentist or surgeon can access your bone. If you have just had a tooth removed, sometimes your gums are left alone or they may be re-shaped for you to have your best result. Then your bone is re-shaped to allow the implant to be placed. If you are already missing a tooth, then a space for the implant needs to be made for the implant to go into. If your tooth was just removed, then the hole your tooth came out of is re-shaped for the implant to fit into. The implant replaces the root of your tooth, but it is not exactly the same shape.

At this point, either your gums will be closed up over the implant to heal and allow your bone to fuse with the implant, a process called osseointegration, or it will be closed around a temporary abutment piece and allowed to heal. Closing your gums completely over the implant keeps bacteria out of the area better, however, the temporary abutments can allow for your gum tissue to heal into a better shape along with the bone healing. Sometimes, the temporary abutments can have temporary crowns on them for aesthetics. Your dentist or surgeon will discuss which option will be best for you.

I have a very reliable patient, my own mother, who I placed my very first implant in just after I started my practice. I thank her for allowing me to write and talk about her and her dental care and to use her as an example. She lost a tooth when I was in high school and had a bridge placed back then. Well, her bridge failed because she got a cavity under the back tooth of the bridge. Food was always catching under it and it was nearly impossible for her to keep it clean. Instead of just doing a root canal on her back tooth and replacing her bridge, we put in two separate crowns and replaced the missing tooth with a dental implant. She was not a candidate for a temporary crown on her implant, so her gums were closed completely over the implant. She chose to be awake for the procedure, and yes, she was still numb for it. The actual placement of the implant she described as just noise and a bit of vibration. When the numbness wore off, it felt like half way between a pizza burn and a Dorito injury. So not painful, but a bit annoying.

Now for healing. As your dental implant heals, your bone will fuse with it and it becomes part of you in a process called osseointegration. It is very important to thoroughly clean the area while your implant is healing to prevent infection. An infection can prevent your bone from fusing to the implant. How long this takes will depend upon your bone. In some bone, this can be as little as 12 weeks. In other bone it can take nine months to a year. Most implants fall in the

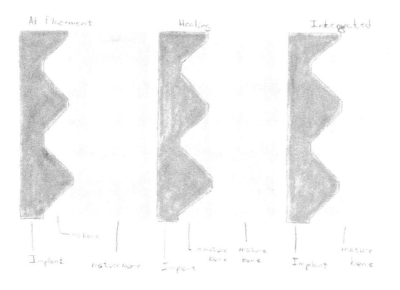

time frame of three to six months. Your mandible, the lower jaw, usually heals faster than your maxilla, your upper jaw.

Once the implant has fused with your bone, an impression will be taken of the area and a crown made for you. There are two options for crowns, cemented or screw retained. There are benefits to each. The cemented has solid material all the way around for better aesthetics, however, the cement can be difficult to remove and can irritate your gums. Also, if anything need to be changed about the crown in the future, it will need to be cut into to remove with at least an access hole drilled into it or possible completely cut off and a new crown made. Cemented crowns are cemented to the abutment connector that goes through your gums in your mouth, after the abutment is attached to your implant. The abutment attaches to the implant with a screw that is tightened to a specific tightness, called torque, to hold it in place. Screw retained crowns are attached all as one piece to the abutment that connects to your implant and have an access hole made into them. Screw retained crowns are not cemented in your mouth. The abutment and crown are screwed onto your implant all as one, and then the access hole is filled. You do not need to worry about the cement irritation to your gums and these can be easily removed in the future if needed, but the access filling may wear or pick up stain over time, just like a filling in a natural tooth. I prefer screw retained so that cement does not irritate your gums, however, due to the necessity of an access hole, may not be an option for everyone.

If you were wondering, my mother originally had a cement retained crown, however, about three years ago, she broke her implant crown, and completely broke the tooth behind it off below the gum line. I have changed her crown out to a screw retained crown and we are working on replacing the tooth behind it. She takes care of her implant and crown the same as any of her other teeth and eats more confidently than she ever had with her bridge.

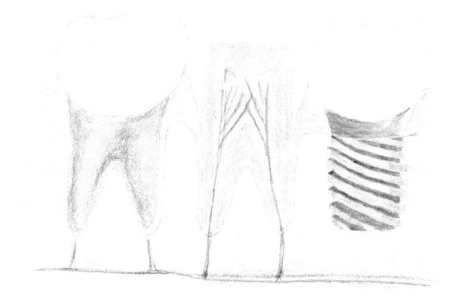

    Now for the variations possible. First, either you are already missing a tooth or you need to have a tooth removed. If you are missing a tooth, and the area has healed, great, you are most likely ready to start. Your bone may need to be re-shaped or added to with grafting. Sometimes this can be done when the implant is placed; sometimes it needs to be done first. The same can be necessary if your tooth is being removed, although it is more likely that you will need bone added when your tooth is freshly removed. If you have a tooth that needs to be removed, sometimes it is possible to put in your implant on the same day, but sometimes you will need to heal after the tooth is removed. Needing time to heal is more likely if your tooth has an infection around it or if your bone is not healthy around it. Sometimes, even if the implant cannot be put in the same day that the tooth comes out but you need to have bone added, that may be able to be done on the day the tooth is removed. If you have other reasons for delaying having your implant placed on the same day as your tooth is removed, having a bone graft placed at the time of extraction can make your bone more ideal for later.

There are variations in healing time. The bone of your maxilla, your top jaw, takes longer to heal than your mandible, your lower jaw. This will cause variation in how long you will need for you bone to fuse with your implant and therefore how long before you have your definitive crown.

Of course, all of the variables specific to you will be reviewed with you at your consultation and examination as well as throughout your treatment.

Maintenance and care

Yes, you do have to take care of your dental implant, just like you need to take care of your teeth. While you cannot get a cavity in a dental implant the way you can in your natural teeth, you still have to take care of the gums around the implant and your other teeth as well. Taking care of the gums is best done by keeping the implant clean. You can still get gingivitis, inflammation of the gums, or peri-implantitis, an infection in the gums around your implant, if you do not clean your implant.

Gingivitis and peri-implantitis are caused by bacteria. Gingivitis is inflammation and is reversible by removing the bacteria. The area will usually look red and irritated and may bleed when brushing and flossing. Peri-implantitis is the same as periodontal disease around your teeth, just around your implant. Peri-implantitis is an infection between your gums and your implant that causes your bone and gum tissue to detach from the implant. As this is the same infection as periodontal disease, it has all the same complications: bone loss, possible implant loss, increased risk of cardiovascular disease, increased risk of heart attacks, increased risk of strokes, increased risk of diabetes, increased risk of Alzheimer's disease, etc. There are whole text books and courses on periodontal disease and peri-implantitis for dentists. I will be working on a guide just like this to translate all of that information for my patients after I have finished this implant book. If you already have periodontal disease on other teeth, you are at increased risk of the infection spreading to your implant and need to be extra vigilant with your home care.

So, how do you take care of your implant. First, the big don'ts. Do not do anything to your dental implant that could break a tooth. The crown of your dental implant is the same materials as a crown on your natural teeth, and is made to mimic your natural tooth structure as closely as possible. Therefore, something that can break your tooth can also break your implant crown. Do not chew ice, avoid grinding your teeth, do not eat rocks, and avoid being kicked in the mouth by a horse. Yes, that has happened to one of my patients. If you did not guess it already, the horse won.

Now how to take care of the implant. You can eat any normal food unless advised otherwise by your dentist. This is most likely if you have a temporary crown on your implant or right around the time when the implant is put in or the crown put on. You will need to clean it, just as you clean your other teeth. You need to clean the biting/chewing surface, the cheek/lip side, the tongue side, and in-between your teeth and your implant. The chewing, cheek/lip side, and the tongue sides are easy, brush them. You can use either a manual or electronic tooth brush, whichever works best for you. If you need help deciding, speak with your dentist or dental hygienist and they can help you to pick out which is best. The key with brushing is to be thorough but gentle. Angle the bristles of the brush so that you sweep out under the edge of your gums, and then sweep across the other surfaces of the tooth to remove all of the plaque and food debris. You do not need to scrub. Scrubbing is for tile and grout, sometimes the wheels of your car, but not for teeth and not for dental implants. Think of your implant and teeth as the world's finest hardwood floors and your gums as the most expensive cabinets. So you angle your broom to get the dust bunnies from under the overhang of the cabinets and gently remove them with little wiggles of your broom, then gently but thoroughly sweep across the floor. Now use your tooth brush on your teeth and implant.

Then take care of the areas between your implant and adjacent teeth. There is more than one way to do this. The simplest is floss, when done correctly; floss is an excellent tool to clean in-between. Take your length of floss and, using as slight sawing motion, go through the tight spots. Hold the floss against the side of your implant crown so that it wraps around it a bit and slide up and down, getting below the gums. Do the same for the tooth next to it and any other teeth that you want to keep. Remember to slide down below the gums as far as the floss will go, but do not force it or snap it or you can cut

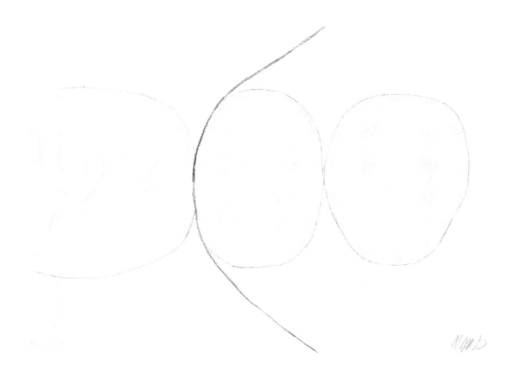

your gums.

There is an alternative flossing technique that works for implants, but not for teeth. Take your floss and put it between your implant and tooth, same as above, then come across on the tongue side and put the floss through on the other side of your implant so that it warps around on the tongue side of your implant with the ends sticking out on the lip/cheek side. Cross the ends in front of your implant then slide up and down and shimmy back and forth. Think of an old fashioned belly dancer doing the dance of many veils. She has removed on of her veils, has it wrapped around her tush, and shimmies it back and forth and up and down. This works well and cleans both sides of your implant at the same time.

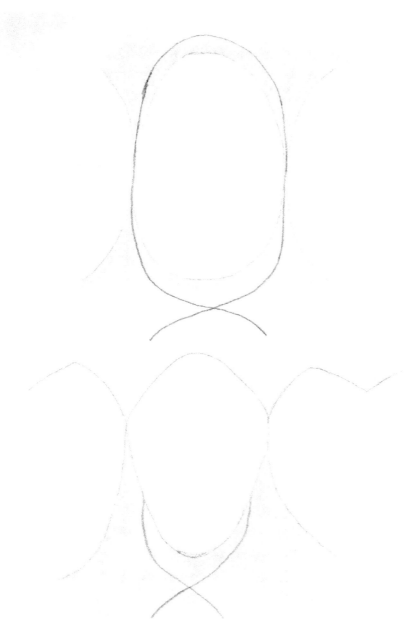

There are also alternatives to floss. So no, you do not have to floss, but you still need to clean between your teeth. There are two main alternatives: water irrigation systems and interdental brushes. Water irrigation, most well-known being the Waterpik brand, use a stream of water to wash out between teeth and implants and under the edge of your gums. For single tooth implants like yours, you can use either the continuous flow irrigator or the interrupted pulse irrigators, although the continuous stream have more uses than just between your teeth and the interrupted pulse irrigators are limited to just the in-betweens. Interdental brushes have a few options. There are end tuft brushes that look like a regular brush with just one or a few tufts of bristles at the end. This small tuft allows you to push the bristles between your teeth. There are interdental brushes that look similar to a pipe cleaner on a stick. These are also pushed between your implant and adjacent tooth. There is also a mechanical tooth brush, the Rotadent, which has a pointy brush tip that is registered as an interdental cleaner as well. The very very thin bristles reach between your teeth and your implant to clean the area. Please note that Rotadent brushes can only be bought through dental offices, although the replacement brush heads are available online. Exactly which of these options is the best for you, your implant, and your teeth is best discussed with your dentist and/or dental hygienist. They will help you to select which of these will be best and easiest for you while effectively cleaning and caring for your implant.

Of course, you will still need regular cleanings at your dentist's office as well, for both your implant and your other, natural teeth. Right after your implant is placed, these may be increased in frequency, until you are able to keep it clean at home, then you will return to your regular routine cleanings.

Remember, you do have to clean your implant, just like you need to clean your teeth, if you want to keep it.

Single dental implants are the closest you can get to having your own tooth back. You clean it like a tooth, eat with it like a tooth, and speak with it like a tooth. Once it is in place, most people think of their dental implant as just like any other tooth.

A Few Missing Teeth

If you are missing a few teeth, or soon will be, but the rest of your teeth are fine, then dental implants are a great replacement for you. There are several options for people who are missing a few teeth, because there are several ways to be missing a few teeth. If you are missing a single tooth from several areas, then you would best be served by several individual single tooth implants. If you are missing two teeth right next to each other, then your restoration options with implants include both single and individual implants or implants that have crowns connected to each other, or you may have one implant

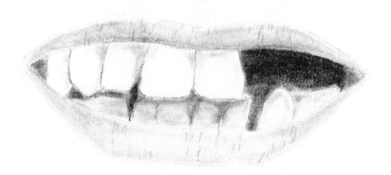

placed with a crown made to look like the two missing teeth together.

The best option for your particular area will be discussed with your dentist or surgeon at your consultation and examination. If you are missing three or more teeth in a row, then you have the option of a bridge, technically a fixed partial denture, which is attached to the dental implants, or possibly replacing the missing teeth with individual implants. Again, the option that is best for you will be discussed at your examination and consultation.

Implant consultation and examination

Before having dental implants placed, you will need to have a consultation and examination with your dentist and/or surgeon. If you are already missing teeth, great, some of your healing has already begun. If you have teeth that need to be removed, then this is done first. Sometimes your dental implants can be put in on the same day as your teeth come out, sometimes your bone will have to heal first, either because of infection or needing to reshape or add to the bone for ideal implant placement. Whether you have teeth present or not, you may also need some work done to re-shape or improve the health of your gums and bone in the area. These will be discussed with you at your consultation.

At your consultation, expect a visual examination of the area as well as some form of X-ray, often a CT scan. The visual exam is to determine the health of your gums and to assess aesthetic and sizing factors for your restoration. The x-rays and/or CT scan are used to determine the health of your bone as well as size and angle of placement of your dental implants. Your dentist or surgeon will discuss with you their findings and if you will need to have any other work done in the area, such as adding bone with a bone graft or re-shaping your gums for better aesthetics and cleanliness.

Your consultation will also cover some of the variations about dental implants. Implants in the maxilla, your top jaw, often take longer to heal than implants in the mandible, your lower jaw. Your exact time frames will be reviewed with you. If you still have teeth that need to be removed, sometimes your implants can be placed on the same day as your teeth come out. Sometimes your bone will need to heal first. Sometimes you can have a temporary replacement restoration attached to your implants on the same day as your implants are put in; however, this depends upon your bone health. Sometimes your gums will need to be closed over the implant and restorations done later. Again, these variables will be discussed with you at your consultation where what is best for you will be determined.

Though there are many variables, as every mouth and every patient is different, there are many things that are the same with dental implants being placed. What I have written here is the usual process and I will mention some of the more common variations as they come up.

Dental Implant Placement

Dental implants replace the root of your tooth in your bone. An attachment piece, called an abutment, comes through your gums to attach your restoration to your implant. Then your restoration goes on top, either a bridge or individual crowns depending upon your treatment needs.

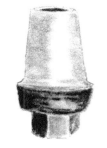

If you have already had your teeth removed, then a small incision is made in your gums so that your dentist or surgeon has access to your bone. If you are having teeth removed on the same day as your implants are being put in, then sometimes your gums are not changed at all, sometimes your gums will need slight modification for ideal placement.

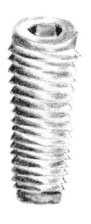

When your dentist or surgeon has access to your bone, a space is made for the implant to go into. If you had teeth removed on the same day, the hole your tooth came out of will be re-shaped slightly. While dental implants replace the roots of teeth, they are not the exact same shape as the root of your tooth, so some re-shaping is necessary.

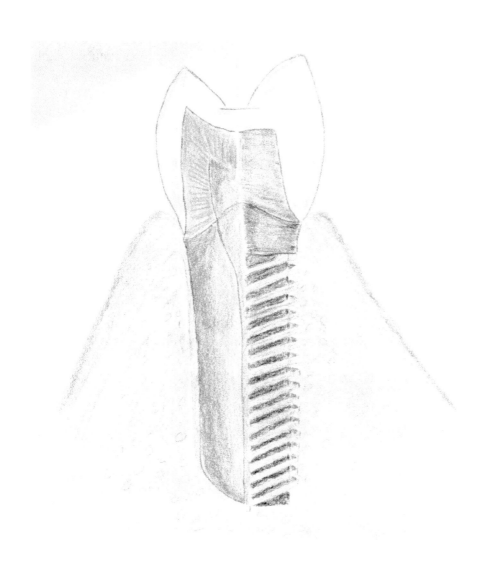

At this point, either your gums will be closed over your implants with a few stitches or temporary abutments will be placed and your gums closed up around them. Your bone is then allowed to heal. During this healing time, your bone fuses with your dental implants and the implant becomes a part of you in a process called osseointegration. Closing your gums completely over the implants keeps bacteria out of the area better, decreasing infection risk; however, placing the temporary abutments allows your gums to heal into a nicer shape while your bone heals at the same time. Some temporary abutments will also allow you to have a temporary bridge or crowns put onto your implants while you heal. Which options are available to you will be discussed with your dentist or surgeon.

Now for the healing phase. It takes some time for your bone to fuse to your implants and the implant to become part of you. It is very important to thoroughly, but gently keep the area clean while you are healing to prevent infection. An infection can prevent your bone from fusing with your implant. Exactly how to best keep the area clean while you heal will be discussed with you as you progress through treatment.

Once your implants have fused with your bone, your definitive restoration, either a bridge or individual crowns, will be made for you. An impression of the area will be taken, then your restorations custom made for you. The abutment, a connector between your implant and your restoration that comes through your gums, will be placed and the restoration attached to it. Depending upon your restoration, either the restoration will be attached to the abutments at the lab when it is made or it will be cemented onto the abutment in your mouth. There are benefits and detriments to each type of restoration and which is best for you will be discussed with you.

The restorations that are attached to your abutments at the lab, also called screw retained, have an access hole in them that will be filled with tooth colored filling material once everything is in place. These provide easier access if your restoration ever needs to have something about it changed, such as if you choose to change the normal tooth shaped restoration to permanently look like a fang because you have landed a life-long acting position as a vampire. It also provides easier access if the restoration ever needs to be removed if you have trouble cleaning it. The drawback of the screw retained restoration is that the filling material can pick up stain, just like a filling in your natural teeth. Screw retained restorations are not cemented in your mouth, and so, you do not have to worry about the cement irritating your gum tissue.

The cemented restoration allows for better aesthetics because it does not have screw access holes. These are also sometimes the necessary restorations due to the positioning of your bone. These restorations are much more difficult to remove if you ever need to have them taken off later, often needing to be cut off and completely replaced instead of being able to be repaired. They also have the possibility of the cement irritating your gums around the restoration if any excess remains after the restoration is placed.

Please note that anything that can break a natural tooth can also break your implant restoration, because the restoration is made out of the same materials as crowns and bridges for natural teeth and is designed to be as close to natural teeth as possible. So, in the event that you happen to break your implant restoration, for example, by being kicked by a horse, then a screw retained restoration would be easier to remove than a cement retained restoration.

Maintenance and care

Yes, you do still have to clean your teeth and your dental implants. While you cannot get a cavity in your implant restoration, like you can in natural teeth, you still have to take care of your gums and bone around the implant, which is best done by keeping your implants clean. You can still get gingivitis, inflammation of your gums, or peri-implantitis, an infection between your gums and implant, if you do not keep them clean.

Gingivitis and peri-implantitis are caused by bacteria. Gingivitis is inflation of your gums and is reversible by removing the bacteria. Gingivitis usually makes the area look red and irritated and may bleed when brushing and flossing. Peri-implantitis is the same infection as periodontal disease around your teeth; just this is around your implants. Peri-implantitis is an infection between your implant and your gums that causes your bone and gums to detach from your implant. As this is the same infection as periodontal disease, it has all of the same complications: bone loss, possible implant loss, increased risk of cardiovascular disease, increased risk of heart attack, increased risk of stroke, increased risk of Alzheimer's disease, etc. There are whole text books and courses on periodontal disease and peri-implantitis for dentists. I will be working on a guide just like this to translate all of the information for my patients after I have finished this implant book. If you already have periodontal disease on your natural teeth, you are at increased risk of the infection spreading to your implants and need to be extra vigilant with your home care.

So, how do you take care of your implants? First, the big don'ts. Do not do anything to or with your dental implant that could break a tooth. The restoration on your dental implants is made of the same materials as a crown or bridge on your natural teeth, and they are made to mimic your natural tooth structure as closely as possible. Therefore, anything that can break your natural tooth can also break your implant restoration. Do not chew on ice. Avoid grinding your teeth. Do not eat rocks. Avoid being kicked by a horse. Yes, that has happened to one of my patients. The horse won.

Now, how to take care of your implants. You can eat any normal food unless advised otherwise by your dentist. This is common if you have had a temporary restoration put on. You then will need to clean your implants, just as you will your other teeth. You need to clean the biting/chewing surface, the lip/cheek side, the tongue side, and in between our implants and between your teeth. The chewing, cheek/lip, and tongue sides are easy; brush them. You can use either a manual or electronic tooth brush, whichever works best for you. The key is to be thorough but gentle. Angle the bristles so that you sweep out under your gums edge. Then sweep across the tooth surfaces. You do not need to scrub. Scrubbing is for tile and grout. Think of your implants and your teeth as the world's finest hardwood floors and your gums as the most expensive cabinets. Your brush is your broom. You want to show off your floors without damaging your cabinets, so you angle your broom to get the dust bunnies out from under the cabinet overhang and gently remove them with little wiggles, then gently but thoroughly sweep across the rest of your floors. Do the same for your implants and your teeth.

    Now to take care of the places between your teeth and between your implants. There are multiple ways to do this, and which is your best option is best discussed with your dentist or dental hygienist. The simplest method of cleaning the in-betweens is floss. When done correctly, floss is an excellent way to clean in between. If you have individual implants with individual restorations that are not connected to each other, then your flossing will be very similar to flossing individual teeth, which will be described shortly. If you have a bridge on your implants, then it is likely that you will need a special tool to floss under the connected area called a floss threader. The floss threader looks like a large, plastic, sewing needle. Thread the floss into the floss threader's eye, and then use the floss threader to pass the floss under the connected part of the bridge. Once the floss is through proceed as follows for flossing.

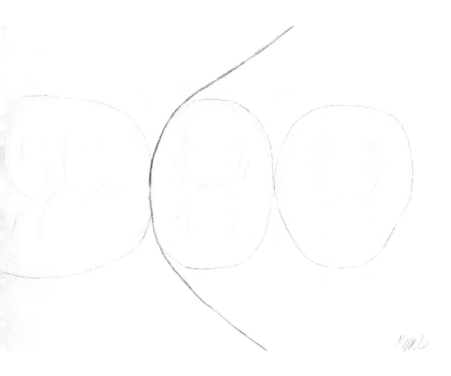

Use a slight sawing motion to move the floss through the tight spot between your teeth and implant, then take your length of floss and hold it against the side of your implant so that it curves slightly around it. Slide the floss up and down gently below the gum line. Do the same for the tooth or implant next to it and any other teeth or implants that you want to keep. If you used a floss threader to pass the floss under a connected area, then slide the floss to the side of the implant, curve around it and gently slide up and down the implant surface below the gum line and up until you touch the restoration. Slide the floss along under the connected portion of your restoration to the next implant and do the same. To remove the floss, simply pull it out from under the connected area and floss normally everywhere else.

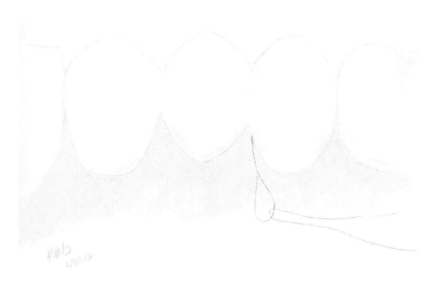

There is an alternative flossing technique that works well for implants, but not for teeth. Place the floss between on one side of the implant as usual, take the other end and wrap it around the tongue side of the implant and come through the other in-between, so that both ends are on the lip/cheek side of the implant. Cross the ends in front of the implant then slide up and down and shimmy back and forth. Think of an old fashioned belly dancer doing the dance of many veils. She takes off a veil, wraps it around her tush and shimmies back and forth and up and down. The image is corny, but you get the picture.

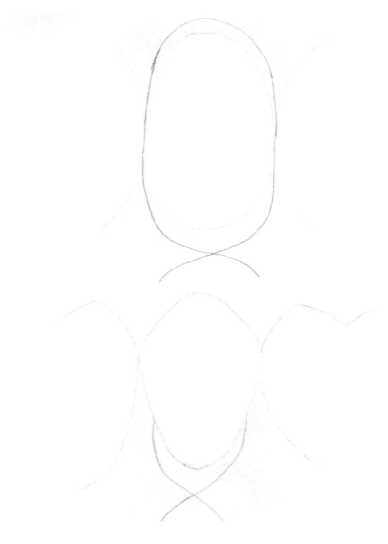

You also have alternatives to floss. So no, you do not need to floss, however, you still have to clean in between. There are two main alternatives: water irrigation systems and interdental brushes, water irrigation systems, the most well-known being Waterpik brand, use a stream of water to flush out any debris and bacteria between teeth and implants as well as under your gums. There are two types of water irrigators, interrupted pulse and continuous stream. The interrupted pulse irrigators can clean between individual teeth, but only the in-betweens. Continuous stream, such as the Waterpik, can be uses for more areas, such as under bridges, with better results in such areas. Interdental brushes come in a variety of styles, and which can work best for you your dentist or dental hygienist can help you to figure out. There are end tuft brushes, which look like a regular tooth brush with only a few tufts of bristles at the end; these allow you to push the bristles between teeth and implants as well as under bridges. There are interdental brushes that look like a pipe cleaner on a stick, which is also slide between teeth and dental implants and under bridges, cleaning with an in and out motion. There is also a mechanical tooth brush, the

Rotadent, which has a pointed brush tip that can clean in between your teeth and implants. Please note that Rotadent brushes can only be purchased through a dental office, however, the replacement heads are available online.

Of course, you will still need regular cleanings at your dentist's office as well, for both your implant and your other, natural teeth. Right after your implant is placed, these may be increased in frequency, until you are able to keep it clean at home, then you will return to your regular routine cleanings.

Remember, you need to clean your dental implants, just like you need to clean your teeth, if you want to keep them.

Dental implants are the closest you can get to having your natural teeth back. You clean them just as you would the same restoration on natural teeth. You eat with them just like natural teeth. And you speak with them, just like natural teeth. Once your implants are in place, most people think of them as being just more teeth, like any other tooth that they have.

Whole Jaw Replacement

Whole jaw replacements are for you if you either do not have any teeth on the top or bottom or both, or if you soon will have all the teeth on top, bottom, or both removed. You are lucky if you fall into

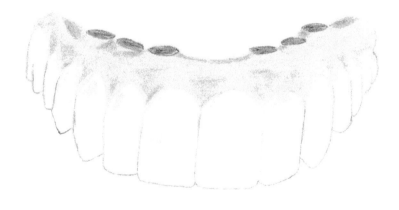

this category because you have multiple options for replacing your teeth with dental implants, more than anyone else.

Your restoration options include having a complete denture that snaps on and off of dental implants, replace every missing tooth with an individual implant and individual crown, and several options in between. Each of the options available to you will be reviewed with you in a moment. The best option for you will be discussed with your dentist or surgeon at your consultation.

Before turning to dental implant replacements, I will briefly review the non-implant options, traditional dentures or gumming it.

Gumming it is just that, using your gums and not replacing your teeth. This is an option, but not a good one. It is difficult to chew and speak. It is also unaesthetic and makes you look older. Over time, your jaw muscles will atrophy and your jaw bone will reduce in size. The one benefit of this option is that the deterioration of your jaw bone is slower than it is when wearing traditional dentures.

Traditional dentures are the standard dentures that have not really changed in a hundred years. They are made of acrylic or other plastics. The top denture stays in place by suction, which depends highly on your jaw shape. The bottom denture stays in place by gravity and muscle control. Most people will use goopy adhesives to help hold the denture in. There is a wide range of quality of materials that affect the durability and longevity of your denture, however all dentures will eventually wear out over time and all of them accelerate the deterioration of your jaw bone so that eventually they will no longer fit and need to be replaced.

In both cases, bone deterioration happens. The bone of your jaw is there to support your teeth. The presence of teeth stimulates the jaw bone and helps to maintain it. When your teeth are no longer present, your body will decide it has better use of the bone materials and takes the bone away for other uses. Dental implants stimulate your bone like teeth, so your bone stays where it is.

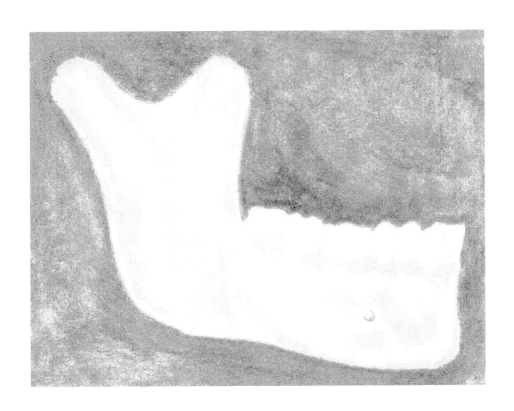

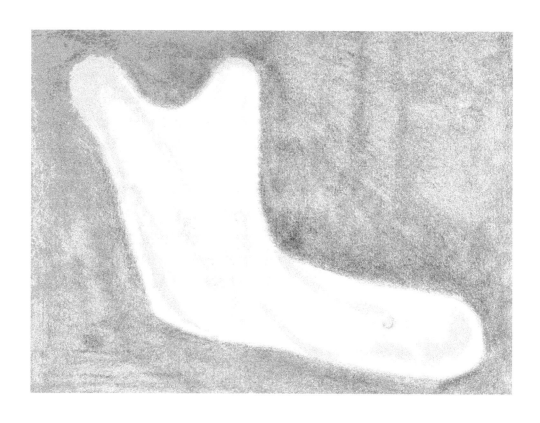

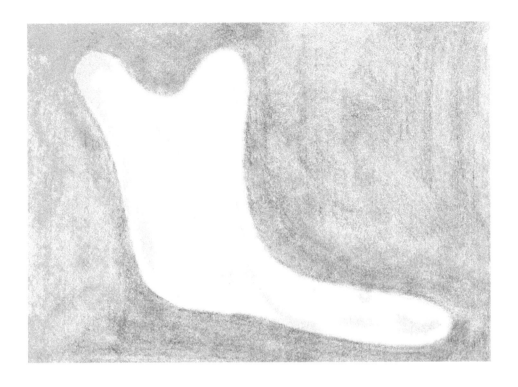

Implant consultation and examination

Before having dental implants placed, you will need to have a consultation and examination with your dentist and/or surgeon. If you are already missing teeth, great, some of your healing has already begun. If you have teeth that need to be removed, then this is done first. Sometimes your dental implants can be put in on the same day as your teeth come out, sometimes your bone will have to heal first, either because of infection or needing to reshape or add to the bone for ideal implant placement. Whether you have teeth present or not, you may also need some work done to re-shape or improve the health of your gums and bone in the area. These will be discussed with you at your consultation.

At your consultation, expect a visual examination of the area as well as some form of X-ray, often a CT scan. The visual exam is to determine the health of your gums and to assess aesthetic and sizing factors for your restoration. The x-rays and/or CT scan are used to determine the health of your bone as well as size and angle of placement of your dental implants. Your dentist or surgeon will discuss with you their findings and if you will need to have any other work done in the area, such as adding bone with a bone graft or re-shaping your gums for better aesthetics and cleanliness.

Your consultation will also cover some of the variations about dental implants. Implants in the maxilla, your top jaw, often take longer to heal than implants in the mandible, your lower jaw. Your exact time frames will be reviewed with you. If you still have teeth that need to be removed, sometimes your implants can be placed on the same day as your teeth come out. Sometimes your bone will need to heal first. Sometimes you can have a temporary replacement restoration attached to your implants on the same day as your implants are put in; however, this depends upon your bone health. Sometimes your gums will need to be closed over the implant and restorations done later. Again, these variables will be discussed with you at your consultation where what is best for you will be determined.

Though there are many variables, as every mouth and every patient is different, there are many things that are the same with dental implants being placed. What I have written here is the usual process and I will mention some of the more common variations as they come up.

Dental implant options

       Implant retained removable dentures

This option is a denture that snaps on and off of dental implants. The implant retained removable denture gives you much more security than traditional dentures and may allow you to have reduced flanges and less coverage of the roof of your mouth. Flanges are the parts that cover over your gums along the sides of your jaw.

First, a bit of

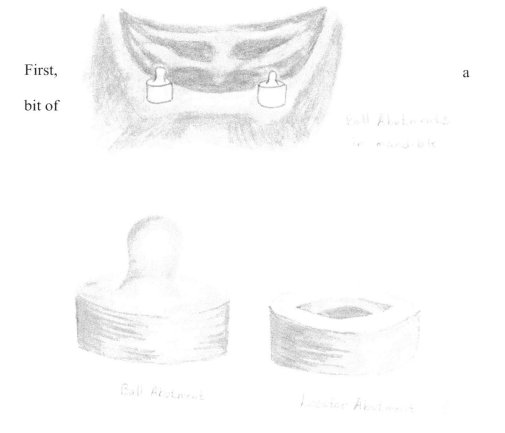

information about dentures. Traditional dentures replace all of the teeth within a jaw, either the maxilla, your top jaw, or the mandible, your bottom jaw. Of course, you can have dentures on both the top and bottom as well.

The similarities between the dental implant retained dentures and traditional dentures is that both are removable, meaning that you take them out to clean the dentures and to clean your mouth. They are both usually made of acrylic or other plastic materials, which do wear out over time in both cases.

The difference between traditional dentures and implant retained dentures is that the implant retained dentures have implants in your jaw and attachments in the denture that help hold them in place, instead of just suction to your gums for the top or gravity for the bottom as it is for traditional dentures. Because of the additional hold, an implant retained denture is much more secure than traditional dentures.

Another difference is that you will need to clean your dental implants. How to care for your implant retained denture and your implants will be covered later in the chapter.

Some people use these as transitional restoration before moving into a non-removable restoration such as a hybrid bridge, which is covered next.

Hybrid bridges

Hybrid bridges are a midway between removable implant retained dentures and full jaw reconstruction with crowns and bridges.

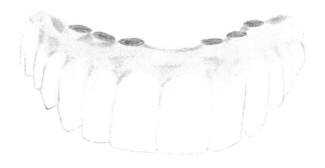

You do not take the hybrid bridge out; however, a dentist can remove it when needed.

For you, it is a large bridge that goes around the whole jaw, replacing all of the teeth in that jaw.

Why would a hybrid need to be removed? There are several reasons. One, the most common, is for cleaning of your implants, especially if you are having difficulty maintaining them yourself and have started to develop peri-implantitis, which will be reviewed further on in the section on cleaning and maintenance. Another reason would be repairs or sometimes replacement of worn teeth, dependent upon the materials used to make the hybrid bridge.

Hybrid bridge prostheses can be made of several materials, and which option is right for you will best be discussed with your dentist, this is just an overview of the options available.

The first option is all acrylic with attachment ports that are usually metal and filled with either acrylic or composite resin once it is in place. This option is usually used as a long term temporary restoration while you are healing, especially when this restoration is put in the same day as your implants are put in. It has the advantage of being highly modifiable and easily repaired, however, it is not as strong as the other options and will wear out faster and can break easier.

The second option is acrylic denture teeth and gums attached to and surrounding a metal bar framework. The bar provides additional strength for the restoration while the acrylic teeth and gums provide ease of repair or replacement. While the bar gives much more strength, the acrylic teeth can eventually wear down and need to be replaced. How long this takes depends upon what you do with your teeth; eating abrasive foods and grinding/clenching your teeth will cause faster wear, just like they do to natural teeth. The bar acrylic combination also requires a larger amount of space between your jaw and the biting surface of the opposite jaw, so it is a better option for people who have already had bone loss, either from periodontal disease of from having worn a denture for a significant amount of time. Otherwise, some of your jaw bone will need to be re-shaped in order to allow room for your hybrid bridge.

The third option is much more like a very large bridge on natural teeth, being made out of the same materials as crowns and bridges for natural teeth. This is either porcelain fused to a metal framework or some of the porcelain/ceramic options such as Zirconia. These are the strongest of the hybrid bridge options; however, repairs to these are a bit more difficult. These have the same wear rate as crowns on natural teeth, so much longer lasting than acrylic teeth options. Being the strongest of the hybrids, they also require the least space for a hybrid between your jaw and the biting surface opposite it, which reduces the need to remove bone to allow your restoration to be placed.

Full jaw reconstruction with individual implants

Full jaw reconstruction is replacing every individual tooth with individual implants or a few bridges when individual replacement is not an option due to your anatomy. Each implant is restored with a single

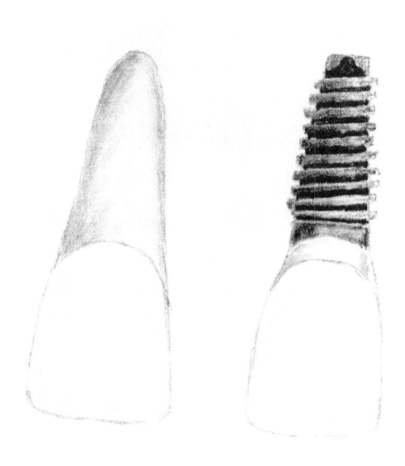

crown or a few bridges just as if you were having every individual natural tooth crowned.

The full jaw reconstruction option requires the greatest number of implants, up to one per tooth, and the greatest amount of planning and parts. It is therefore the most expensive option. The aesthetics of this option is highly dependent upon the contours of your bone and gums, which may need to be modified, either removing some for smoothness or adding some where you are deficient. This option, of all full jaw replacement options, does require the least amount of space between your jaw and

the biting surface of the opposite teeth , so it is the least likely to require the removal of bone, other than for aesthetics. You are actually more likely to need bone grafting to add bone where you need more.

The individual implant restoration option is not removable for you and difficult to be removed by your dentist, sometimes requiring it to be cut to remove it, therefore, it is the most difficult option to repair, however, it is also a strong option and when any repairs are necessary, only those areas that need to be repaired are removed. The restorations are made of the same materials as crowns for natural teeth, so anything that can break a crown on a natural tooth can break these restorations. In other words, chewing on rocks is not advisable; neither is eating handle bars and being kicked by a horse. Yes, I have had a patient kicked by a horse. The horse won.

Implant placement.

Implants are placed very similarly for all of these options. The difference comes with the quantity and location of the implants as well as the attachment pieces that are put onto them. There is also some variation in timing, depending upon your options.

First, you are either in need of removing your teeth or have already had your teeth removed. If you are already missing your teeth, great, some of your bone healing has already started. When you do not have teeth, a small incision is made so that your gums can be moved out of the way to access your bone. If you have just had your teeth removed, sometimes, your gums will be left alone, or they may be re-shaped for you to have the best result. Then your bone is re-shaped to allow your implants to be placed. If you teeth are already missing, a space is made in your bone for your implants to go into. If your teeth were just removed, sometimes the holes left by your tooth roots will be reshaped, sometimes those are filled with bone graft and allowed to heal and new, better placed spaces are made. The implants replace the roots of your teeth, but they are not the exact same shape as your roots, so some modification is usually necessary.

    At this point, either your gums will be closed over the implants to heal and allow your bone to fuse to your implants or your gums will be closed up around temporary abutments, a connector piece that comes up through your gums, and allowed to heal. Closing your gums completely over the implants keeps bacteria out better; however, the temporary abutments allow your gums to heal into shape along with your bone healing. Having temporary abutments can often allow for a temporary restoration to be attached to your implants if you are having a non- removable restoration placed. This gives your aesthetics and function while you heal. Your dentist or surgeon will discuss which option is best for you.

Now for healing. As your dental implants heal, your bone will fuse with the implant in a process called osseointegration and your implant becomes part of you. It is very important to thoroughly clean the area while you are healing to prevent infection. An infection can prevent your bone from fusing to the implant.

When your bone has fused to your implants, work can begin on your definitive restoration. The process for each of the restoration options are described below.

Implant Retained Removable Dentures

For this option, you most likely have been wearing a removable denture. This is either the denture you had before your implants were placed, or a temporary denture that was made for you to wear while healing. Take the time to really look at your current denture. Ask yourself if there is anything that you specifically like about it? Do you like the color of the teeth? What about the color of the gums? How about the size and shape of the teeth? Anything that you like, make a note of it, same for anything you would change about it. Now is the time to make such changes, so please discuss these with your dentist when you are starting out.

The restoration process for you will start with at least one set of impressions. There are a variety of techniques for making implant retained dentures, so the specifics will vary by which way works best for your dentist. I even vary my techniques dependent upon my patient, so I will describe the classic method, which even that has a few variations within it. I will note the variations for you when we get to them.

The classic method starts with an initial alginate impression. Alginate is an impression material that is used to make a model of your mouth. It is usually lightly flavored, but often a bit chalky, and it starts like pudding and sets like jello. The model that is made from this is used to make a custom impression tray that fits you and only you. The custom tray impression is much more accurate.

With the custom tray impression, there are several impression materials that can be used. Some taste good, some taste nasty, but your dentist will use the one that works best for them and will give you the best result. These impressions usually take a little longer to set than the alginate initial impressions, but the custom tray makes it more comfortable.

The next step is called a wax rim, or occlusion record. Most often, this is done using wax that is customized to your mouth in the general shape of where your teeth are going to be. This is mostly a reference for work that will be done in the lab. Measurements and markings are made into the wax, such as where the middle of your face is, where your eyes align, making sure your teeth will be horizontal instead of slanted. There is a variation that depends upon your mouth. Sometimes the wax rims can be attached to your custom trays. Sometimes the wax rims need to be separate, making them a separate step and sometimes a separate appointment. The next step is trying in your teeth, so all of the things that you like and things you want to change about your current teeth should be discussed at this point or earlier.

Tooth trial is your next step. Your actual denture teeth will be set up in a moldable, usually wax, material to replicate your gums. Please note that this moldable material is often a little bright in color. This is to make sure that all of it is cleaned off before the next step in the lab. This is the appointment where you get to change things. Do you like the color, size, shape, and position of your denture teeth? Of course, your dentist will check the fit, bite, and speech positioning, but you are the one who gets to decide if you want a gap between your front teeth or not, if you want your teeth to be fresh from the orthodontist straight or do you prefer some slight, more natural variations? If you have someone whose opinion is valuable to you, it would be a good idea to bring them along to this appointment. This is your opportunity to have a say in how your smile will look. Your teeth will come in with an initial setup. They will be moved from there to your preference.

There is a variation at this point. If your dental implants have not been placed yet, this wax setup will be used as a guide for the implants to be placed. If you already have your dental implants, and they have healed, then your implants will be uncovered, meaning that any gum tissue over the implant will be removed, you will not need that gum tissue any more as a temporary healing abutment will likely be placed to keep your gums from growing over the implants again. This space is where your attachment abutments will go through your gums. A pickup impression would be completed with your wax setup so that the lab can plan for your attachments to be in your denture. Alternative timings for this impression include during your final impression and after the initial processing of your denture.

When you have approved of your wax setup, then it is sent to the lab for processing. The processing replaces the wax with acrylic or plastic. In some cases, a metal framework will be imbedded into your denture for added structural stability when needed. The lab may put the implant attachments into the denture at this point or your dentist may do this in the office when you are present. Both options work and each has advantages that your dentist can review with you.

If the implant attachments were not placed by the lab, then they will be done at the office. For this, your denture has already been processed and is ready for you. Your healing abutments will be removed and your implants uncovered. Your implant attachments will be placed onto them and torqued into place. Torqueing, tightening them to a specific tightness, keeps your abutments stably attached to your implants. A place for the denture attachments will have been left in the gum side of the denture. Your dentist may need to modify this for the best fit for you. The denture attachment is then placed onto your implant attachment. Pickup material is then placed into the denture so that everything bonds together and the denture is placed into your mouth and over your implants and the attachments. Once the pickup material has set, the denture is removed from your mouth and it is cleaned and polished. Cleaning removes all excess pickup material and double checks the security of the denture attachments. A similar process is done when using an impression with the pickup at the lab, but on your models.

Please note that there are some variables for removable implant retained dentures that I have not yet covered. First, there are variations in numbers of implants that are needed. Of course, your dentist or surgeon will discuss with you what your specific needs are. The usual minimum requirements are at least two implants on the lower jaw and at least four implants on the top. The reasons for the difference in minimum numbers are due to the mechanics of chewing and the different densities of bone in your top jaw versus your lower jaw. A second variation is in the need for a retaining bar attached to your implants. Some people will need a bar and some will not. The bar provides additional security for your denture, variation of attachment points, and allows the implants to be braced against each other for better force distribution. Your dentist will discuss the need for a bar. The third variation is the attachment types. There are ball and O-rings, locators (which look like a clothing snap), clips that attach to a specific bar shape, as well as pins that go through a bar. Each has advantages and disadvantages and your dentist will review which is best for you.

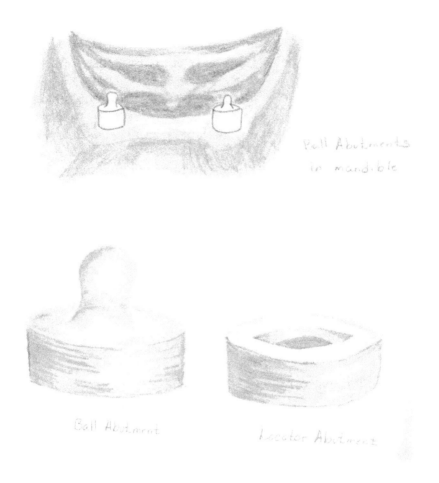

Now that you have your implant retained removable denture, you will need to know how to maintain it and your implants. This section could be called, yes; you still need to clean your teeth. When you are out and about, you can use some quick touchups when you need to, such as swishing with water or mouthwash or lightly brushing over your denture with an extra soft tooth brush. When you are at home and are fully cleaning your implant retained denture and your implants, you can do a more thorough and complete cleaning. Start by taking out your removable teeth. These can be cleaned similarly to any regular denture. Using warm water, rinse and gently brush off any debris. There are special cleaning pastes, similar to tooth pastes, made just for use on dentures. These do not have the abrasives in regular tooth pastes, which can take the polish off of the denture. You can also use the various denture soaks to aid in cleaning. Please note that some of the attachment pieces require specific cleansing soaks, and your dentist will let you know if your implant retained denture attachments have this specification.

Once your denture has been cleaned, keep it either moist, in a zip top baggie or in water until you will be wearing it again. This is for your comfort. Most modern denture materials can dry out without any harm to the material; however, if they are dry when you put them in, it will feel as though it is sucking all the moisture out of your mouth. That feeling can last for a few hours. If you clench or grind your teeth at night, or did with your natural teeth, it will be best to keep the implant retained denture out at night to decrease the wear on the denture as well as any other restorations and teeth that you have. There are other reasons to keep the denture out at night, such as allowing your saliva to bathe your gums, that your dentist can review with you for your best health and maintenance.

Now to take care of your implants and attachments. Yes, you do have to clean your implants, so keep the brush and floss. While you cannot get a cavity in your implant restoration, like you can in natural teeth, you still have to take care of your gums and bone around the implants, which is best done by keeping your implants clean. You can still get gingivitis, inflammation of your gums, or peri-implantitis, an infection between your gums and implant, if you do not keep them clean.

Gingivitis and peri-implantitis are caused by bacteria. Gingivitis is inflation of your gums and is reversible by removing the bacteria. Gingivitis usually makes the area look red and irritated and may bleed when brushing and flossing. Peri-implantitis is the same infection as periodontal disease around your teeth; just this is around your implants. Peri-implantitis is an infection between your implant and your gums that causes your bone and gums to detach from your implant. As this is the same infection as periodontal disease, it has all of the same complications: bone loss, possible implant loss, increased risk of cardiovascular disease, increased risk of heart attack, increased risk of stroke, increased risk of Alzheimer's disease, etc. There are whole text books and courses on periodontal disease and peri-implantitis for dentists. I will be working on a guide just like this to translate all of the information for my patients after I have finished this implant book. If you had periodontal disease on your natural teeth, you are at increased risk of the infection spreading to your implants and need to be extra vigilant with your home care.

Start with brushing the implants and attachments. You can use either a manual or electric tooth brush, whichever works best for you. The key is to be thorough but gentle. Angle the bristles so that the sweep out under your gums, and sweep across all other surfaces that you can reach. You do not need to scrub. Scrubbing is for tile and grout, sometimes the wheels of your car, but not for teeth and not for dental implants. Think of your implants as the world's finest hardwood floors and your gums as the most expensive cabinets. You want to show off the floors without damaging the cabinets, so you angle your broom to get the dust bunnies from under the overhang of the cabinets and gently remove them with little wiggles of your broom, then gently but thoroughly sweep across the floor. Now use your tooth brush on your implants. If your implants are all individual, meaning not attached to each other with a bar, it is likely that brushing may be all you need to do, as long as you can reach around all sides of every implant. To supplement brushing, if you are unable to clean with a regular tooth brush all areas of every implant, you will need to floss, use a water irrigation system, or an interdental brush.

    Take your floss and put it on one side of your implant, then come across on the tongue side and put the floss through on the other side of your implant so that it wraps around on the tongue side of your implant with the ends sticking out on the lip/cheek side. Cross the ends in front of your implant then slide up and down and shimmy back and forth. Think of an old fashioned belly dancer doing the dance of many veils. She has removed on of her veils, has it wrapped around her tush, and shimmies it back and forth and up and down. This works well and cleans both sides of your implant at the same time.

There are also alternatives to floss. So no, you do not have to floss, but you still need to clean the areas you cannot reach with a brush. There are two main alternatives: water irrigation systems and interdental brushes. Water irrigation, most well-known being the Waterpik brand, use a stream of water to wash out between and around implants and under the edge of your gums. There are two types of water irrigation systems, continuous stream and interrupted flow. In your case, the continuous stream is likely to be the better option. Interdental brushes have a few options. There are end tuft brushes that look like a regular brush with just one or a few tufts of bristles at the end. This small tuft allows you to push the bristles between and around your implants. There are interdental brushes that look similar to a pipe cleaner on a stick. These are also pushed between your implants. There is also a mechanical tooth brush, the Rotadent, which has a pointy brush tip that is registered as an interdental cleaner as well. The very very thin bristles reach between your implants to clean the area. Please note that Rotadent brushes can only be bought through dental offices, although the replacement brush heads are available online. Exactly which of these options is the best for you and your implants is best discussed with your dentist and/or dental hygienist. They will help you to select which of these will be best and easiest for you while effectively cleaning and caring for your implants.

If you implant retained denture attaches over a bar connected to your implants you will need to clean around the implants and under the bar. Floss is an excellent way to do this. If your bar has ends extending beyond your back most implants, slide the floss under one end and use a gentle back and forth motion to slide all the way to the side of your back most implant. Curve the floss around the side of your implant and slide up and down on that side. Use a floss threader to bring the floss under the bar between implants. A floss threader looks like a giant plastic sewing needle. Put one end of the floss into the eye of the threader and use the threader to pull the floss under the bar. If you want, you can wrap the floss around your implant and shimmy up and down to clean both sides at the same time, then release the end of the floss under the back end of your bar and slide across under the bar to the next implant. Repeat this process across under your bar until you

reach the other end.

Your bar may have some space under it, between the bar and your gums. If this is your case, an interdental brush will probably be easier and faster than floss. There are two main types of interdental brushes. The first looks like a regular brush but with only a few tufts of bristles at the end. The other looks like a pipe cleaner on a stick. Slide the brush carefully under the bar, then using an in and out motion, brush all areas of the underside of the bar and the sides of your implants.

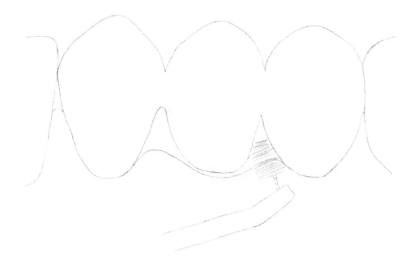

An alternative to floss or the interdental brushes is a water irrigation system. There are two types of irrigation systems, continuous stream or interrupted pulse. The continuous stream works better for the bar.

As for any home care routines, your dentist or dental hygienist can review with you what is the best way for you to clean and maintain

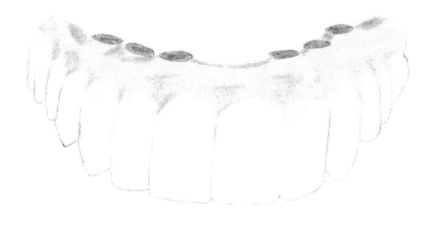

your mouth, implants, and denture.

Hybrid Restorations

Hybrid restorations are half way between a removable implant retained denture and complete jaw reconstruction. You do not remove the hybrid, but a dentist can if needed.

There are some variables for hybrid restoration, largely in the materials used, which were reviewed previously. All of the materials have advantages and disadvantages. The best option for you will be discussed with you by your dentist. Just as a review options for materials include full acrylic, acrylic teeth over a metal bar, and porcelain with a metal or ceramic framework or full ceramic, also called zirconia.

You also have some additional options regarding timing. Often, you can have a temporary restoration put on the same day as your implants are put in, even if it is the same day as your teeth are removed. This temporary restoration is one that you do not take out, so you will care for it and clean it in your mouth. There are specifics of that care that will be reviewed with you by your surgeon or dentist that are mostly because of the implants having just been placed and your gums needing to heal. If you are having a temporary hybrid put in on the same day as your implants are put in, then you will start with impressions to make models of your mouth first. These will vary slightly depending upon if you have teeth or not before your implants are put in, but all of them are to record the shape and location of you jaw so that your implants can be placed properly and a temporary restoration can be ready for you. Once your implants are in place and stable, then the temporary restoration will be attached to them. This usually uses special temporary abutments, parts that come through your gums to attach the restoration to your implants that are designed just for use with a temporary restoration. The temporary hybrid bridge will, most likely, be held in place with screws that have access holes at the abutments. These will be filled with acrylic or composite (tooth colored filling material) so that your dentist can remove the temporary when your implants have fully healed. The temporary restoration splints your implants together to distribute chewing forces, which allows the implants to still fuse with your bone while having a restoration that you do not take out. Cleaning of your temporary will be reviewed a little further ahead as cleaning of all hybrid bridges use similar techniques.

There are a few precautions with temporary hybrid bridges. First, because your implants have been newly placed, you will likely be given an eating plan to slowly acclimate your mouth to eating and chewing foods with your new hybrid bridge and implants. I have presented here an example plan; however, yours will vary based upon your bone health at the time when your implants are put in.

Example eating plan

Time	Food type	Example food
First week	Very soft and mushy	Scrambled eggs, oatmeal, mashed potatoes, yoghurt, soup, protein shakes, smoothies
Second week to three months	Soft foods that can be cut by a fork – stewed, steamed, or braised foods that are moist and easy to chew	In addition to above, soft fish, turkey and chicken, meatloaf, soft pasta, rice, canned/cooked vegetables, bananas, avocados, canned fruits
Foods to avoid while healing	Foods that require tearing or biting with front teeth, hard crunchy foods	Bread, bagels, all nuts and seeds, salads, dried fruits, apples, raw vegetables, pizza, steak, tough meats, gum, ice, etc.

While you have your temporary restoration, think of it as the prototype of your definitive restoration. What do you like about it? What would you change? Do you like the color, size, and shape of the teeth? How does your bite feel? If you have someone whose opinion you value, ask them as well. Remember, this is the stage that you can make changes. You will have your temporary restoration for a while and will likely be seeing your dentist periodically while you wear your temporary. These periodic visits allow for some adjustments to be made to your temporary while you wear it. It is with your temporary that your bite is double checked and perfected for your comfort and long term stability.

Your definitive hybrid bridge is largely based upon your temporary hybrid. So the starting point for your definitive hybrid bridge is often an impression of your temporary. This ensures that your bite is accurate to the comfortable position that your temporary is in. Please note that I am using the term definitive hybrid instead of permanent for a reason. Anything that could break your natural teeth has the potential to break your definitive hybrid restoration, which would be removed and repaired or replaced. If you want to make significant changes, such as deciding to change the teeth to be fangs for a lifelong acting position as a vampire, a new hybrid can be made for you with fangs. If you lose the ability to use your hands and are no longer able to clean your hybrid yourself, then it can be removed for professional cleanings. So there are a variety of reasons for not saying permanent and using definitive instead.

There are several options for materials for your definitive hybrid bridge. These include acrylic over a metal framework, porcelain over a metal framework, porcelain over a ceramic framework, and fully ceramic hybrid bridges. There are advantages and disadvantages to each of these and your dentist will recommend which is your best option.

The process of making your definitive hybrid restoration is similar to making your temporary. Several impressions will be taken, some with your temporary in place, some without the temporary, and some of these may have been done along the way and while making your temporary. Your definitive restoration is made for you, then, when your bone has healed and is ready for it, your temporary restoration is removed and your definitive hybrid restoration is put in place. The definitive restoration will have access holes for it to attach to your implants. These access holes are filled, usually with tooth colored filling material called composite resin. Then you smile, eat, and speak with it, knowing that it stays in place.

Now that you have your hybrid bridge, you need to take care of it and keep it clean. Anything that can break your natural teeth can break your hybrid; therefore, it is best to avoid chewing on rocks and being kicked by an angry horse. That may sound silly, but I have had patients kicked by horses before. It damages them and their teeth. If you have a temporary hybrid, especially if it was put in the same day as your implants, then your dentist or surgeon will instruct you on any additional precautions while you are healing.

Yes, you do have to take care of your hybrid bridge and your implants. While you cannot get a cavity in a dental implant the way you can in your natural teeth, you still have to take care of the gums around the implants. Taking care of the gums is best done by keeping the implants clean. You can still get gingivitis, inflammation of the gums, or peri-implantitis, an infection in the gums around your implants, if you do not clean your implants.

Gingivitis and peri-implantitis are caused by bacteria. Gingivitis is inflammation and is reversible buy removing the bacteria. The area will usually look red and irritated and may bleed when brushing and flossing. Peri-implantitis is the same as periodontal disease around your teeth, just around your implants. Peri-implantitis is an infection between your gums and your implants that causes your bone and gum tissue to detach from the implants. As this is the same infection as periodontal disease, it has all the same complications: bone loss, possible implant loss, increased risk of cardiovascular disease, increased risk of heart attacks, increased risk of strokes, increased risk of diabetes, increased risk of Alzheimer's disease, etc. There are whole text books and courses on periodontal disease and peri-implantitis for dentists. I will be working on a guide just like this to translate all of the information for my patients after I have finished this implant book. If you had periodontal disease on your teeth before they were removed, you are at increased risk of the infection spreading to your implant and need to be extra vigilant with your home care.

Cleaning and caring for your hybrid bridge and implants is a two-step process. To start, clean the teeth part of the hybrid. The simplest way to do this is to brush it, just as you would brush your teeth. Brush all parts of the hybrid that you can reach with a soft or extra soft brush. You can use a mechanical or manual tooth brush, which ever works best for you. You do not need to scrub. Scrubbing is for tile and grout, sometime the wheels on your car, but not teeth or implants. Then you will need to clean under the hybrid and around your implants. There are several ways to clean under the hybrid including flossing, interdental brushes, and the use of water irrigation systems. Your dentist will help you to learn which way will work best for you.

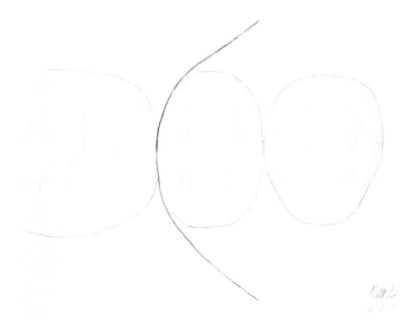

Floss is an excellent way to clean below the hybrid bridge. If your hybrid bridge has ends extending beyond your back most implants, slide the floss under one end and use a gentle back and forth motion to slide all the way to the side of your back most implant. Curve the floss around the side of your implant and slide up and down on that side. Use a floss threader to bring the floss under the hybrid between implants. A floss threader looks like a giant plastic sewing needle. Put one end of the floss into the eye of the threader and use the threader to pull the floss under the hybrid. If you want, you can wrap the floss around your implant and shimmy up and down to clean both sides at the same time, then release the end of the floss under the back end of your bar and slide across under the bar to the next implant. Repeat this process across under your hybrid until you reach the other end.

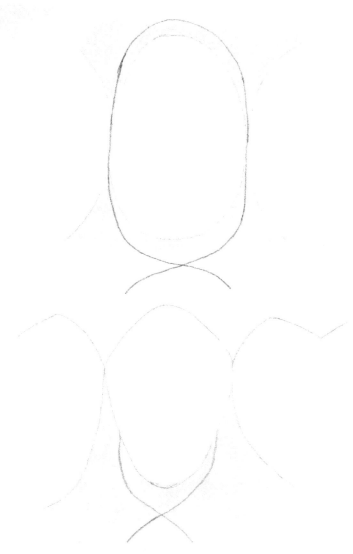

Your hybrid bridge may have some space under it, between the hybrid and your gums. If this is your case, an interdental brush will probably be easier and faster than floss. There are two main types of interdental brushes. The first looks like a regular brush but with only a few tufts of bristles at the end. The other looks like a pipe cleaner on a stick. Slide the brush carefully under the hybrid, then, using an in and

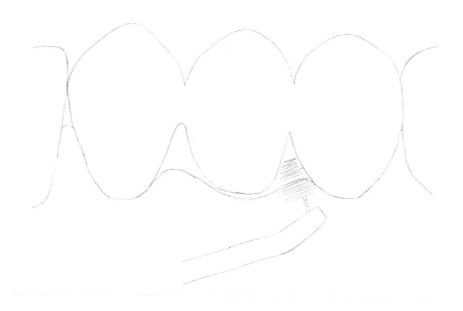

out motion, brush all areas of the underside of the hybrid bridge and the sides of your implants.

An alternative to floss or the interdental brushes is a water irrigation system. There are two types of irrigation systems, continuous stream or interrupted pulse. The continuous stream works better for hybrid bridges.

Full Jaw Reconstruction

Full jaw reconstruction replaces your teeth with individual implants with individual crowns or possibly a few bridges. This is the most complicated option as each implant for each missing tooth is planned for individually , however, it also gives you the complete ability to treat your implants just like teeth, brushing them, flossing between them individually, and of course, eating, and speaking with them. This option is also the most expensive of the full jaw replacement options as it has the greatest number of implants, up to one per tooth replaced, and is the most likely option to require gum tissue and bone grafting to reshape and replace your gums and bone for function and aesthetics.

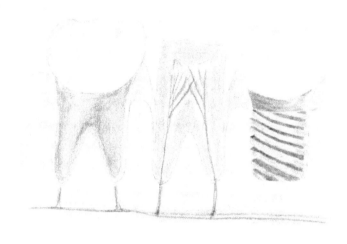

For full jaw individual implant reconstruction you will have several phases to your treatment. First your teeth, if you presently have them, will need to be taken out. Some or all of your implants may be put in when your teeth are removed, however, it is also possible that you may just have bone or gum tissue augmentation completed at this time as well, depending upon the condition of your jaw. You will likely need to wear a denture during the healing phases, and you may be asked to keep the wearing of your denture to a minimum, especially if you have had certain types of grafts placed. Your dentist and surgeon will review your specific instructions with you.

If your grafting or tooth removal had to be separate from your implant placement, then you will have a second surgery appointment to place your implants. This is followed by healing time to allow your bone to fuse with your implants. If you are already missing your teeth, then a small incision is made so that your gums can be moved out of the way and your dentist or surgeon can access your bone. If you have just had your teeth removed, sometimes your gums are left alone or they may be re-shaped for you to have your best result. Then your bone is re-shaped to allow the implant to be placed. If you are already missing your teeth, then spaces for the implants needs to be made for the implant to go into. If your teeth were just removed, then the holes your teeth came out of are re-shaped for the implant to fit into. Dental implants replace the roots of your teeth, but they are not exactly the same shape.

At this point, either your gums will be closed up over the implants to heal and allow your bone to fuse with the implants, a process called osseointegration, or your gums will be closed around temporary abutment pieces and allowed to heal. Closing your gums completely over the implant keeps bacteria out of the area better, however, the temporary abutments can allow for your gum tissue to heal into a better shape along with the bone healing. Your dentist or surgeon will discuss which option will be best for you.

While your implants are healing, it is likely that you will be wearing a traditional removable denture or you will have a temporary non-removable hybrid bridge. The hybrid bridge will have your teeth attached to each other like a giant bridge. If you have this option, please look back at the hybrid bridge option for the process and maintenance of this temporary hybrid.

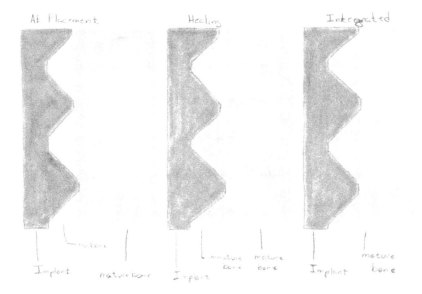

I have a very reliable patient, my own mother, who I placed my very first implant in just after I started my practice. I thank her for allowing me to write and talk about her and her dental care and to use her as an example. She lost a tooth when I was in high school and had a bridge placed back then. Well, her bridge failed because she got a cavity under the back tooth of the bridge. Food was always catching under it and it was nearly impossible for her to keep it clean. Instead of just doing a root canal on her back tooth and replacing her bridge, we put in two separate crowns and replaced the missing tooth with a dental implant. She was not a candidate for a temporary crown on her implant, so her gums were closed completely over the implant. She chose to be awake for the procedure, and yes, she was still numb for it. The actual placement of the implant she described as just noise and a bit of vibration. When the numbness wore off, it felt like half way between a pizza burn and a Dorito injury. So not painful, but a bit annoying.

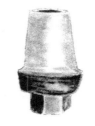
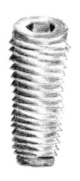

Once your bone and your implants are fused, then your restorations are started. If you are wearing a denture, it is possible that your gums may have healed over your implants. If this is the case, the gum tissue just over your implants is removed as part of shaping your gums for your restorations. I am using restorations in the place of repeatedly typing crowns and/or bridges. Impressions abutments are placed onto your implants and a series of impressions are taken. Your impression abutments (sometimes called copings) are removed and either your temporary restoration or healing abutments are put back on while an initial set of shaping restorations are made.

Your shaping restorations are used as a trial run of your final restorations while also allowing modifications to perfect both your bite and the shape of your gums and teeth. You will likely have several appointments to check your tissues and bite while you wear your shaping restorations to allow for these modifications

When your bite and gums are stable and in their best positions, another series of impressions are completed to make your definitive restorations. Your definitive restorations will be made of the same materials as crowns and bridges for natural teeth, and need to be treated accordingly. When your definitive restorations are ready for you, your shaping restorations will be removed and your definitive restorations placed.

Now that your full jaw reconstruction restorations are in place, you will need to take care of them and your implants. While you cannot get a cavity in dental implants the way you can in your natural teeth, you still have to take care of the gums around the implants. Taking care of the gums is best done by keeping the implant clean. You can still get gingivitis, inflammation of the gums, or peri-implantitis, an infection in the gums around your implant, if you do not clean your implant

Gingivitis and peri-implantitis are caused by bacteria. Gingivitis is inflammation and is reversible buy removing the bacteria. The area will usually look red and irritated and may bleed when brushing and flossing. Peri-implantitis is the same as periodontal disease around your teeth, just around your implants. Peri-implantitis is an infection between your gums and your implants that causes your bone and gum tissue to detach from the implants. As this is the same infection as periodontal disease, it has all the same complications: bone loss, possible implant loss, increased risk of cardiovascular disease, increased risk of heart attacks, increased risk of strokes, increased risk of diabetes, increased risk of Alzheimer's disease, etc. There are whole text books and courses on periodontal disease and peri-implantitis for dentists. I will be working on one just like this to translate all of the information for my patients after I have finished this implant book. If you had periodontal disease on your teeth before they were removed, you are at increased risk of the infection spreading to your implant and need to be extra vigilant with your home care.

So, how do you take care of your implants. First, the big don'ts. Do not do anything to your dental implant that could break a tooth. The crowns on your dental implants are the same materials as a crown on your natural teeth, and are made to mimic your natural tooth structure as closely as possible. Therefore, something that can break your teeth can also break your implant crowns. Do not chew ice, avoid grinding your teeth, do not eat rocks, and avoid being kicked in the mouth by a horse. Yes, that has happened to one of my patients. If you did not guess it already, the horse won.

Now how to take care of your implants. You can eat any normal food unless advised otherwise by your dentist. This is most likely while you have a temporary hybrid or while you have the shaping temporary crowns. You will need to clean all parts of your implants and your crowns. You need to clean the biting/chewing surface, the cheek/lip side, the tongue side, and in-between your implants. The chewing, cheek/lip side, and the tongue sides are easy, brush them. You can use either a manual or electronic tooth brush, whichever works best for you. If you need help deciding, speak with your dentist or dental hygienist and they can help you to pick out which is best. The key with brushing is to be thorough but gentle. Angle the bristles of the brush so that you sweep out under the edge of your gums, and then sweep across the other surfaces of your implants to remove all of the plaque and food debris. You do not need to scrub. Scrubbing is for tile and grout, sometimes the wheels of your car, but not for teeth and not for dental implants. Think of your dental implants as the world's finest hardwood floors and your gums as the most expensive cabinets. So you angle your broom to get the dust bunnies from under the overhang of the cabinets and gently remove them with little wiggles of your broom, then gently but thoroughly sweep across the floor. Now use your tooth brush on your implants.

Then take care of the areas between your implants. There is more than one way to do this. The simplest is floss. When done correctly, floss is an excellent tool to clean in-between. Take your length of floss and, using as slight sawing motion, go through the tight spots. Hold the floss against the side of your implant crown so that it wraps around it a bit and slide up and down, getting below the gums. Do the same for the implant and crown next to it and any other implants that you want to keep. Remember to slide down below the gums as far as the floss will go, but do not force it or snap it or you can cut your gums.

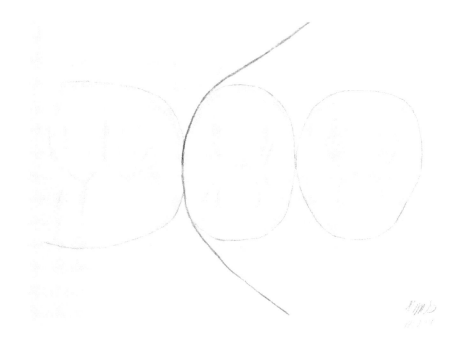

There is an alternative flossing technique that works for implants, but not for teeth. Take your floss and put it between your implants, same as above, then come across on the tongue side and put the floss through on the other side of your implant so that it warps around on the tongue side of your implant with the ends sticking out on the lip/cheek side. Cross the ends in front of your implant then slide up and down and shimmy back and forth. Think of an old fashioned belly dancer doing the dance of many veils. She has removed on of her veils, has it wrapped around her tush, and shimmies it back and forth and up and down. This works well and cleans both sides of your implant at the same time.

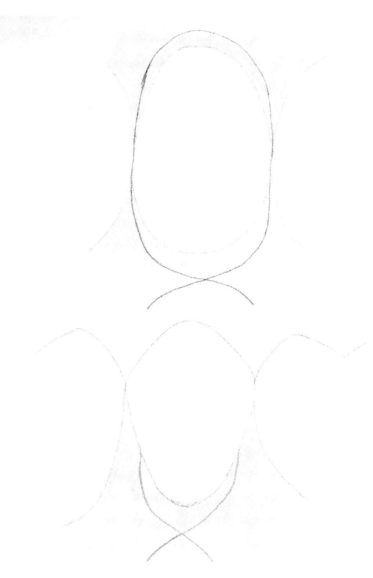

There are also alternatives to floss. So no, you do not have to floss, but you still need to clean between your implants. There are two main alternatives: water irrigation systems and interdental brushes.

Water irrigation systems, most well-known being the Waterpik brand, use a stream of water to wash out between teeth and implants and under the edge of your gums. For single tooth implants like yours, you can use either the continuous flow irrigator or the interrupted pulse

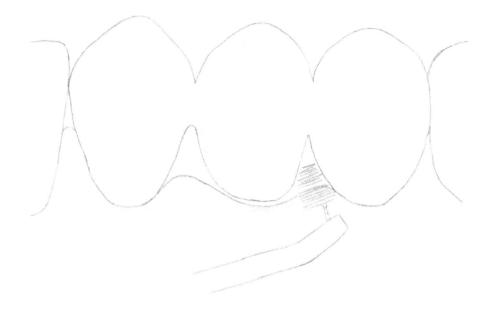

irrigators, although the continuous stream have more uses than just between your teeth and the interrupted pulse irrigators are limited to just the in-betweens. Interdental brushes have a few options. There are end tuft brushes that look like a regular brush with just one or a few tufts of bristles at the end. This small tuft allows you to push the bristles between your implants. There are interdental brushes that look similar to a pipe cleaner on a stick. These are also pushed between your implants. There is also a mechanical tooth brush, the Rotadent, which has a pointy brush tip that is registered as an interdental cleaner as well. The very very thin bristles reach between your implants to clean the area. Please note that Rotadent brushes can only be bought through dental offices, although the replacement brush heads are available online. Exactly which of these options is the best for you, your implants, and your teeth is best discussed with your dentist and/or dental hygienist. They will help you to select which of these will be best and easiest for you while effectively cleaning and caring for your implants.

Remember, you do have to clean your implant, just like you need to clean your teeth, if you want to keep it.

Other considerations and topics

Dental implants in orthodontics

Sometimes dental implants are used for other purposes besides replacing your teeth. The main other use is in orthodontics.

Orthodontics is the process of straightening your teeth and jaw bone; most people know at least a bit about braces and many have had them. Braces work by pushing and pulling your teeth to move them in your jaw. Implants can aid in this.

There are two main implants used. The first is the regular root type of implant, the same as used for replacing your teeth. The second type are called temporary anchorage devices, or TADs. The regular root type implants are used when a strong, long term force is needed to move your teeth as these implants are much stronger and stay in better and longer than the TADs. The TADs are much smaller and much more temporary, sometimes being put in and taken out and possibly placed in a different location throughout treatment. In either case, they are used to provide an additional point to pull and push against and are often used to accelerate your orthodontic treatment compared to other traditional treatment methods. If you will need implants during your orthodontic treatment, your orthodontist will discuss this with you.

Who would not benefit from dental implants?

This is just a note on patients who will not do well with dental implants or may need to delay their dental implant treatment.

To start with, if your natural teeth are fine, you are not missing any, and no teeth are un-restorable, then you most likely will have no need for dental implants, because you have nothing to replace. If your teeth are otherwise fine, but you do not like the color, size, shape, position, etc. of your teeth, these can all be changed with restorations and possibly orthodontics. You have options besides taking them out just to have a pretty smile.

If you are allergic to medical titanium, then there is the option of Zirconia ceramic dental implants. Zirconia ceramic implants are still being studied for longevity and durability; however, they are an option for those few people allergic to medical titanium. Zirconia ceramic implants are still very new in the US market and not widely available. There are also some components that are still being worked on and they do not yet have all of the restoration options that traditional titanium implants currently have. The majority of dental implants are made of medical titanium, the same as hip and knee replacements. Restoratively, there are many options for materials, so any one material allergy would not in itself be an issue that would prevent you from replacing your teeth.

If you have a serious medical issue, it does not mean that you cannot have dental implants, but it might mean that you cannot have them right now or your treatment may take longer. Examples of this are: 1) If you are actively undergoing chemotherapy or radiation therapy, take care of that treatment first, and when your oncologist/physician releases you, then look into implants. 2) if you are an uncontrolled diabetic, then it will slow your healing and increase your risk of infection. You will do better, throughout your body, when your diabetes is under control. 3) if you are like my dad (Yes, I have his permission to use him as an example) and you need major heart surgery, get that done first. In this case, if your heart stops working, then your teeth do not really matter at that point. 4) If you are pregnant, your ob/gyn may ask you to delay any elective procedures, such as having an implant put in or restored, until after the baby is born. So take care of any major medical, life threatening issues as they take priority. Other medical issues we can work with your physician to replace your teeth.

The last group of people who would not want dental implants are those who are truly happy missing their teeth. If you like having the gap in your mouth where a tooth was, if you just really like taking out your denture or prefer to just have gums, then stay just the way you are. Yes, there are benefits to having dental implants, such as having a restoration that is as close to having natural teeth as possible, and preservation of bone, better aesthetics and function, but if you do not want them, then I will not force you to have them.

Cost

One of the major concerns that my patients have is the cost of dental implants. Yes, there is an expense to dental implants, however, there is an expense to any replacement for missing teeth. So it is really just choosing which option you want to spend your money on.

As there are several options for tooth replacements, and your total costs will be unique to your situation, I will make some generalizations here, just so that you have some ideas for comparison.

Some dental insurance plans cover dental implants and some do not. Some insurance companies cover parts of implants, but not the whole thing. Some just set a reduced fee for you, but do not pay anything toward the implants. You would have to contact your insurance or your dental office to find out if your particular plan covers dental implants or not. Then, just to complicate the insurance factor, some medical insurance plans will cover parts of the implants, but sometimes medical insurances will only cover these procedures at a specialist's office, such as an oral surgery office. The specifics of your plan would need to be discussed with your dentist to find out what your plan covers. Just remember, it varies by plan, and sometimes changes when plans renew.

So, let's take dental insurance out of the picture so that you can get an accurate comparison of costs. For a single tooth replacement, a dental implant is usually within $300-500 of a three unit bridge, the alternative fixed replacement for your tooth, and the implant has a much longer average lifespan. For full jaw replacement options, the costs vary even more, depending upon your options, how many implants you need and what restoration you choose.

Whether you have dental insurance or not, there are financial options for dental implants. Some dental offices will split up your payments, usually covering what is done on any given day on that day. Procedures that take several steps may be split up step by step. There are also third party financing companies. One that I work with is Care Credit. Care Credit allows you to sign up at home or in the office and is a medical credit card. Care Credit has no interest options. Care Credit is accepted in many offices and can be used for dental, medical, vision, plastic surgery, veterinary care for your pets, and many other medical related treatments. With the low and no interest options, dental implants can be accessible for everyone.

Fear

I know that dentistry can be scary. You have someone working in your mouth, where it is difficult or impossible for you to see what they are doing. Sometimes you are in pain before the work starts. Sometimes you need to have a shot to be numb. I have had patients that have cried in my office even before I saw them. One patient, I did not get to see her until her third time in the office, she was so terrified. We work with patients that are afraid. There are options.

Dentistry has changed a lot over the years. It has changed even while I have been in practice. Digital technologies are making dentistry more comfortable and accurate. Lasers are making it so we do not always need to numb. Ultrasonic cleaners, which actually were developed in the 1950's, make having your teeth cleaned much faster, more effective, and are kinder and gentler to your teeth and gums.

For the very fearful patients, there are sedation options. In my office, I offer nitrous oxide, which many people know of as laughing gas. The oral surgeon that I work with offers IV sedation in his office. IV sedation lets patients sleep through the whole procedure, but they breath on their own and can be woken back up either with medications or, often, by gently shaking their shoulder and telling them to wake up. For medically compromised patients, and those that are just too scared, he can also take patients to the operating room at a local hospital, where they can be completely sedated for surgery. There are options, you just have ask.

New technologies

Dental implants have been around for many years now. I have patients that had their implants placed in the early 1980's, and while I wanted to be a dentist way back then, I knew nothing about dental implants that long ago. These patients' implants are still there and will probably be there for the rest of their lives. But dentistry is ever evolving and there are new technologies that are giving better results faster with more options.

As I already mentioned above about allergies, zirconia ceramic dental implants are becoming available, but are still being studied and developed. Because the implant and the abutment are all one piece, there is a lot more work involved in designing the ideal placement of zirconia implants. Currently these are made similarly to titanium implants in a variety of shapes and sizes, but soon they may be able to custom make the implants for each person individually.

In the grain of everything old is new again are blade style implants. Blade style implants are flat, instead of round like the root form implants that have been pictured throughout this book. Blade style implants used to be all one piece, like the current zirconia ceramic implants and had limitations on the restorations available. The current blade style implants have attachments that fit many of the standard abutments. These are designed for use if you have a very thin jaw bone in the cheek to tongue side direction. The placement technique for these is slightly different from the root form implants because of the difference in shape. Instead of making a round space, a slot is made to slide the implant into.

There are advances being made in the instruments used to place implants, such as condensation burs that compact spongy bone so that implants are more stable faster and can sometimes widen a thin jaw bone without needing to add graft material. There are new technologies that use some of your own growth factors, chemicals that your body makes that speed healing, such as platelet rich plasma (PRP) or platelet rich fibrin (PRF). For these, a small amount of your own blood is drawn up and the growth enhancing components taken from it and put at your implant site. There are even lab made growth factors that can enhance your bone and gum tissue, instead of having to draw blood to use your own.

There are some new attachments and abutments that are giving more patients even more options. One of these is similar to a locator for implant retained removable dentures, except that you cannot take it out and the restoration is more like a hybrid bridge. Your dentist would be able to remove it without having to unscrew the hybrid bridge so no access holes that are filled in afterward.

With many offices becoming entirely digital, there are now digital options for your x-rays and for your impressions. All of the x-rays that you would have in a dental office have digital options, from the regular little ones in your mouth up to the cone beam CT scans that are used for dental implants. The digital radiographs offer enhanced visibility, more information, and much less x-ray exposure for you. Digital impressions use imaging of your mouth to create a three dimensional computer model of your mouth. Some of these use a powder to give a better image, some do not. And sometimes you will have some impressions digitally and some with traditional impression materials.

There is something that is being worked on, the only option that could be more natural than dental implants. Scientists are working on re-growing teeth. It is still very experimental and not available for people yet. So far, they have made something that has all the parts of a tooth in the correct order, but it is not tooth shaped. Will replacing teeth with new, lab grown teeth become a reality? Yes, will it be functional in my life time? I am not sure. It is certainly many, many years before it becomes available, and because these would be natural teeth, they can get cavities and periodontal disease, just like any other tooth.

These and many more technologies will make dental implants faster, safer, more comfortable, and more available to more people as time continues.

Conclusion

Thank you for allowing me to give you more knowledge of dental implants and how they can be the best restoration for you, whether you are missing one tooth or all of them. I truly believe that dental implants are a large part of the future of dentistry and will continue to become more prevalent.

As always, a consultation with your dentist or surgeon will be able to provide you with the best treatment plan to meet your needs and desires. You now have the information to be able to converse with your dentist about dental implants and you will be able to understand if your dentist starts to use technical jargon. There is a dental implant dictionary, with pictures from this book, at the very end for you as well, just in case something comes up you will not have to search for it.

Once you and your dentist have decided which your best option is, you already know the basics of what to expect and how treatment will progress, as well as how to take care of your implants afterward. Remember, you only need to clean the implants that you want to keep.

While I would love to see all of you in my office, I know that Apopka, Florida may be a bit out of your way. There are many excellent dentists that work with dental implants throughout the US and around the world. I recommend starting with your regular dentist that you are already comfortable with. Discuss your options. If your regular dentist does not work with dental implants, then look into local oral surgeons, periodontists, and prosthodontists. These are dental specialty doctors that handle more complex care. If you need additional resources, I recommend your local dental society, the American Dental Association, the American Academy of Dental Implantologists, and the International Congress of Oral Implantologists. While there are many great dentists that are members of these organizations, there are many great dentists that are not, which is why I recommend starting locally and finding a dentist that you are comfortable with.

I wish you happy and healthy smiles for a lifetime.

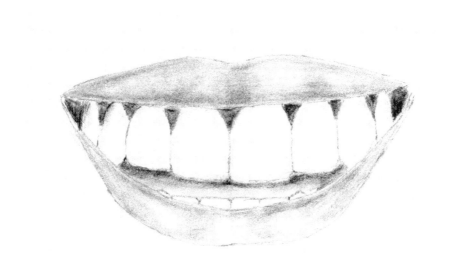

Dental Implant Dictionary

Abutment – a connector that goes between your dental implant and your restoration through the gum tissue

Access hole – a hole in a restoration that allows access into the interior, often for the retaining screw.

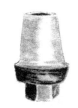

Acrylic - a plastic material that is used to make many types of dental restorations including dentures, temporary crowns, and temporary hybrid bridges.

Adjacent teeth – the teeth next to your dental implant

Aesthetics – how your implant restoration and your other teeth look. May also be spelled esthetics.

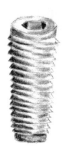

Alginate - an impression material that is used to make a model of your mouth, one of several materials available. It is often used to make study models and for temporary restorations.

Alzheimer's disease – a disease that causes one of several types of dementia. Specifically, this causes memory loss that worsens over time.

Atrophy – deterioration of an area, usually causing reduction in size and may reduce density and quality of structures

Attachment – a part in a removable implant retained denture that allows the denture to snap on and off of dental implants

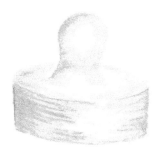
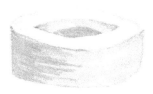

Bell Abutment   Locator Abutment

Average life span – how long, on average, a restoration will last. Being an average, it takes into account the restorations that are not cared for as well as those with excellent care and those that have had unfortunate trauma. Dental implants have one of the longest average life spans of all dental restorations.

Bacteria – germs. You have both good and bad bacteria in your mouth. It is the bad ones that we worry about. The good ones help to protect your mouth from fungi

Bite – both a noun and a verb. The verb means to bring your top and bottom teeth together to touch. The noun is the way your teeth touch when they are together. Do your lower teeth come out in front of your top teeth? Do your top teeth and bottom teeth touch evenly on both sides? This is your bite.

Biting surface – the surfaces of teeth that touch when they are together

Bridge - also called a fixed partial denture – this is a restoration to replace one or more missing teeth that has a connection at each end, either a dental implant at each end or a natural tooth at each end.

Cardiovascular disease – diseases that cause deterioration of your blood vessels (arteries and veins) as well as your heart

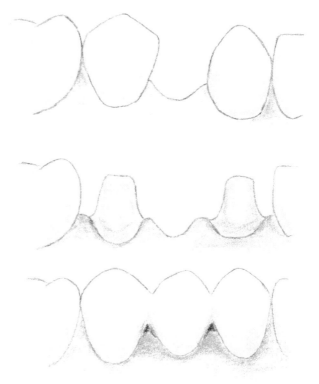

Carries – often called cavities – lesions in your teeth that are caused by bacteria

Cavities - an area of missing tooth structure, a hole in a tooth. These can be caused by wear, acid erosion, abrasion, or bacteria. When caused by bacteria, they are specifically called carries or a carious lesion

Cement – a material that holds a restoration onto a tooth or an abutment

Cemented restoration – a restoration that is held on by cement

Ceramic – a one of several restorative materials available, it is very strong – an inorganic, non-metallic, crystalline material that is used for dental restorations

Complete denture – a denture that replaces all of the teeth on the top or bottom jaw

Composite – tooth colored filling material

Consultation - an appointment with your dentist or surgeon where your treatment options are reviewed with you.

Continuous stream – a type of water irrigation system where the water is sprayed out constantly

Crown - the part of a tooth that you can see, also a restoration that covers or replaces the part of a tooth that you can see

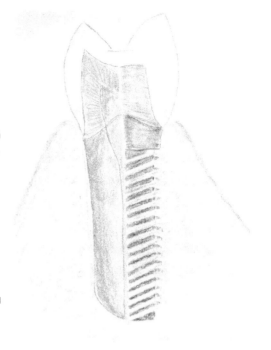

CT scan – a type of x-ray that produces a three dimensional reconstruction of your jaw bone. This is used for planning the positioning of your dental implants within your bone. Also may be called a CBCT, which stands for Cone Beam Computed Tomography

Custom impression tray – a tray used to take an impression of your mouth that has been custom made to fit you and only you.

Definitive restoration – the intended final tooth replacement. These

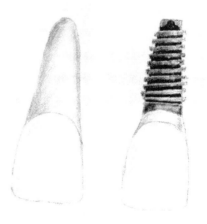

restorations are intended to last as long as you do, however, there are a variety of reasons that it may need to be removed or replaced, and therefore, they cannot be called permanent.

Dental implant – a replacement for the root of your tooth. It goes into your bone and holds an abutment and restoration to replace your tooth or teeth.

Dental restoration- a replacement for your tooth, teeth, or parts of teeth. Also can refer to a crown, filling, or bridge on natural teeth or to a complete or partial denture as well as restorations on dental implants.

Dentist – a doctor that has specialized their care and training to just the mouth and parts of the mouth

Dental Hygienist – a licensed dental professional who specializes in cleaning your teeth and care for the health of your gums, teeth, and surrounding bone.

Dental lab – the place where dental restorations such as crowns, bridges, dentures, hybrid bridges, etc. are made

Denture adhesive – a substance that helps to hold in traditional complete dentures and partial dentures by sticking to the denture and your gum tissue. There are three types, gel, powder, and wafer.

Denture soak – a product used in the cleaning of removable restorations. Typically it is a powder or tablet that is dissolved in water and the removable restoration placed into it and allowed to soak for a set amount of time to aid in removal of food debris and bacteria.

Deterioration - the process of becoming progressively worse. In reference to bone, it includes reduction in size and amount of bone as well as bone density.

Detriment - a cause of harm, damage, or negative consequence

Diabetes – a disease that causes increased blood sugar. Increased blood sugar causes harm to the rest of your body.

Electronic tooth brush – a tooth brush that uses an electric motor to increase motion. The increased motion can aid in cleaning, especially for people who have limited or reduced dexterity of their hands or a care taker who has to clean someone else's teeth

End tuft brush – a type of tooth brush that has one or a few tufts of bristles at the end, usually used to clean between teeth and implants or other hard to reach places

Examination – an appointment where your teeth, gums, and bone are reviewed and evaluated for health and planning of dental implant restorations

Extraction – removal of a tooth

Few missing teeth – when you are missing more than one tooth but less than all of them in a jaw. You may be missing one from several different areas or several teeth in a row.

Fixed - not removable, stays still

Fixed partial denture – the technical term for a bridge - this is a restoration to replace one or more missing teeth that has a connection at each end, either a dental implant at each end or a natural tooth at each end.

Flange – a part of a denture that extends over the gums tissue between the gum and cheek/lip or between the gum and tongue. Provides stability to a denture.

Floss - a string like material that is used to clean the sides of teeth and implants that have adjacent teeth or implants where a brush cannot reach

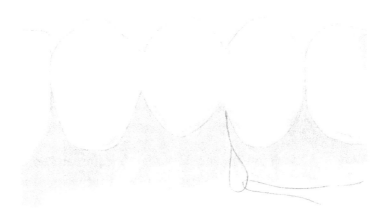

Floss threader – a device used to pass floss under a bridge or bar. Can also be used to pass floss around and under orthodontic appliances. Looks like a large plastic sewing needle

Food debris – food that remains stuck to your teeth or implants and restorations after you have finished eating. This food then feeds bacteria that cause carries, gingivitis, and periodontal disease.

Full jaw reconstruction – replacement of all teeth in a jaw, either maxilla or mandible, possibly both

Function – the use of your teeth, examples being eating and speaking

Gingiva – technical term for gum tissue

Gingivitis – inflammation around a tooth or implant that is caused by bacteria. If allowed to remain, can progress to periodontal disease or peri-implantitis. Gingivitis is reversible if bacteria are removed.

Graft – material that is added to an area that is deficient. This can be bone or gum tissue. Some grafts are taken from other areas of your body or mouth. Some grafts use donated material, some are artificially made in a lab

Gumming it – not a technical term, but used commonly – meaning to go without a replacement for teeth, often used in reference to not wearing a complete denture. Using gum tissue to eat and speak instead of a restoration

Gum line – the line where your gum tissue ends and visible tooth begins

Gums – technically called gingiva – the pink soft tissue around your teeth and over your bone

Heart Attack – sudden lack of blood supply to part of the heart. Can cause death of the affected region of the heart muscle and/or the person

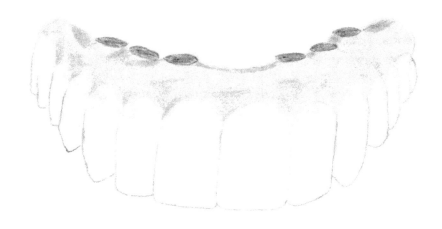

Home care – how you take care of your teeth and implants at home

Hybrid Bridge – a restoration that replaces all of your teeth in a jaw. You do not remove the restoration, however, your dentist can if needed for cleaning or repair.

Implant retained removable denture – a removable complete denture that snaps on and off of dental implants

Impression – a process to make a model of your mouth. This can be done physically using impression materials, such as alginate, polyvinylsiloxane, polyether, or polysulfide, which start soft and mushy and become firm, or can be completed using electronic imaging devices

Impression abutment – a piece that attaches to an implant that comes up through the gums specifically for the purpose of taking an impression to relate the implant's position in your mouth to the lab. Also called an impression coping

Impression coping - a piece that attaches to an implant that comes up through the gums specifically for the purpose of taking an impression to relate the implant's position in your mouth to the lab. Also called an impression abutment

Incision – the process of making a cut in tissue. Can be completed using a

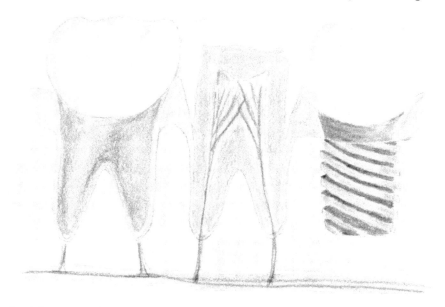

scalpel, laser, or electrosurgey device

Individual implants – implants that the restorations do not connect to each other

Interrupted flow – a type of water irrigation system where the water is sprayed in a start and stop fashion. Best used only between teeth

Implant placement- the process of putting a dental implant into the jaw bone

Jaw – the bone that holds your teeth or dental implants. Top jaw is referred to as the maxilla. Bottom jaw is referred to as the mandible

Long term temporary – a temporary restoration that you will wear for longer than two weeks up to a year

Maintenance - procedures to take care of your restorations and teeth so that you keep them for as long as possible

Mandible – lower jaw

Manual tooth brush – a tooth brush that is entirely moved by hand

Maxilla – top jaw

Metal Bar Framework – a piece of metal that is inside of a restoration to give it additional structural stability and longevity.

Modifiable – able to be changed

Natural tooth – a tooth that you grew

Non-removable – fixed. Cannot be taken out

Normal food – foods that are considered normal to eat, not rocks, ice, bone, sand, forks, etc.

Numb - lack of feeling in an area

Occlusion record – a record for laboratory use in making your restorations that includes how your jaws are positioned compared to each other as well as to the rest of your face and head

Oral Surgeon – a dentist that has specialized in just the surgical components of dental care. May also be called an oral and maxillofacial surgeon

Orthodontics - the process of moving teeth within the bone to straighten them

Orthodontist - a dentist that has specialized in just the movement of teeth to

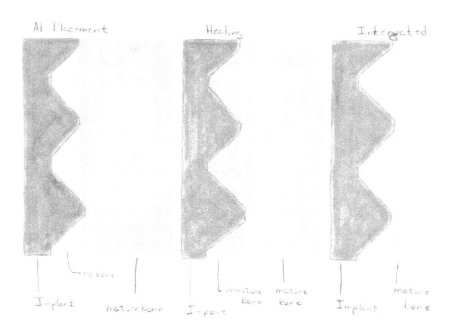

straighten them

Osseointegration – the process of a dental implant fusing to your bone and becoming part of you. Some texts will use osteointegration as an alternative.

Peri-implantitis – an infection around your implant that causes your bone and gum tissue to detach from your implant. This is caused by the same bacteria that cause gingivitis and periodontal disease.

Periodontal disease - an infection between your gums and tooth that causes your bone and gums to detach from your teeth. Also has systemic complications including increased risk of cardiovascular disease, heart attack, stroke, type II diabetes, etc.

Periodontitis – another name for periodontal disease

Periodontist – a dentist that has specialized in the treatment of periodontal disease. May also remove teeth and place implants when done in conjunction with such treatment

Pickup impression – an impression that holds attachments so that the location of implants and abutments can be relayed to the lab in conjunction with the model of the jaw

Pickup material – material that is used to add an attachment into a removable implant retained denture

Plaque - a sticky bacteria film that forms on teeth and restorations. The bacteria in plaque cause carries, gingivitis, and periodontal disease

Porcelain fused to ceramic – a type of restoration material that has a ceramic substructure with porcelain fused to the surface of the ceramic for better aesthetics

Porcelain fused to metal – a type of restoration material that has a metal substructure with porcelain fused to the surface of the metal for better aesthetics

Prosthodontist - a dentist that has specialized in making complex restorations including implant restorations

Prototype – a temporary restoration that is used as a trial run restoration, to test your bite and confirm aesthetics and function

Radiograph – technical term for an x-ray

Removable partial denture – a removable restoration that replaces some of the teeth in a jaw but not all of the teeth in a jaw. May have one or several teeth

Removable replacements – a tooth replacement restoration that can be taken in and out of the mouth. Includes removable partial dentures, complete traditional dentures, and implant retained dentures

Restoration – a replacement for part or all of a tooth

Retaining screw- a screw that holds the abutment of an implant restoration to the implant

Saliva - the liquid that lubricates your mouth and aids in chewing, also called spit

Screw retained restoration – a restoration that is connected to the abutments so that the retaining screw holds both on together

Single missing tooth – when only one tooth is missing

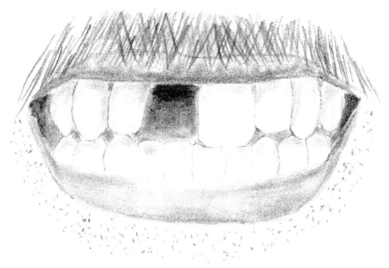

Single tooth dental implant – a dental implant that replaces only one tooth

Shaping restoration- a temporary restoration that is placed in order to improve the shape of the gum tissue. May be adjusted over time, often a long term temporary restoration

Standard of care – considered the minimum to which care needs to be kept up to. Offering dental implants to eligible patients is the standard of care

Study model – a model of your mouth that is used in the planning portion of your treatment. Components of treatment may be made from this

TAD = temporary anchorage device – a small temporary implant that is used in orthodontics

Temporary Abutment – a connector between an implant and a temporary crown that comes up through the gum tissue. Sometime these may not be connected to a crown and only come through the gum tissue for shaping

Temporary anchorage device – a small temporary implant that is used in orthodontics, also referred to as a TAD

Temporary Crown - a crown restoration that is worn temporarily while healing and another, definitive crown is being made

Time frame – the length of time that it takes for something to occur

Tooth root – the portion of the tooth that is normally within your bone, may become exposed by periodontal disease. The portion of the tooth that is replaced by a dental implant

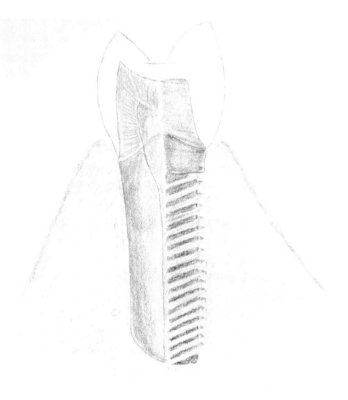

Tooth trial – a step in the fabrication of some restorations, where teeth or tooth representatives are set in a moldable material so that they can be moved to your preference and best function

Torque – tightening to a specific tightness to prevent loosening

Traditional Denture – a denture that replaces all teeth in a jaw without implant attachments, also called a complete denture or traditional complete denture

Transitional restoration – a long term temporary restoration that is used while in progress toward a different type of restoration, can sometimes be a definitive restoration for another person

Unaesthetic – not nice in appearance

Vigilant – keeping careful watch for possible danger or difficulties

Visual Examination – and examination that looks directly into your mouth to determine the health of your visible tissues (teeth, gums, and tongue)

Water Irrigation System – a cleaning device that uses a spray of water to clean between teeth and implants and under restorations

Wax rim – a step of fabrication of some restorations that uses wax to relay information about your jaw and face to the lab

Whole jaw restoration – replacing all of the teeth in a jaw with an implant restoration

X-ray – also called a radiograph, an image of the hard tissues of your teeth and jaw

Zirconia – a type of ceramic that is both aesthetic and strong, used for restorations

Acknowledgements

Special thanks to Dr. Ronald J. Trevisani, for placing implants for me and taking excellent care of my patients, as well as being the first to teach me about dental implants, even before I became a dentist.

Thank you to Leo, for making beautiful crowns.

Thank you to Dr. Jack Jones, D.M.D, Dr. Boyd Welsch, D.D.S., Dr. Matthew Dennis, D.D.S, Dr. Ernest Lado, Jr, D.D.S, and Dr. I. Jack Stout, PhD. for being the best training faculty I have ever had.

Last, but not least, a huge thank you to my family, for supporting me through all of my training, and for being my example patients for so many things.

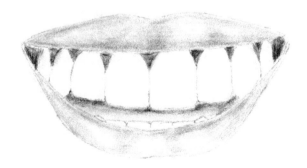

About the author

Dr. Katrina M. Schroeder is a general dentist in Apopka, Florida. She has been in practice since 2006, seeing patients of all ages and with mouths in all conditions. Dr. Schroeder provides care for all aspects of dentistry, including fillings, cosmetic dentistry, veneers, whitening, and, of course, dental implant restorations.

She has studied dental implants extensively and strives to make sure that all patients that would benefit from implants are aware of the options available to them. Dental implants are the passion that drives her practice. Dr. Schroeder is dedicated to making sure that her patients know their options for their care and what the benefits and detriments of each option are, so that they can make the best decisions for their own health and happiness.

Dr. Schroeder completed her Doctor of Medicine in Dentistry (D.M.D) at the University of Florida College of Dentistry and her Bachelors of Science at the University of Central Florida in Biology with a Chemistry minor and University Honors.

When not with her patients, Dr. Schroeder enjoys spending time with her family, reading (usually about dentistry) and biking. She participates in several charity running events each year. Her hobbies include writing, painting, and restoring antique and classic cars.

$20 Examination and Consultation

This is an offer for anyone who has read through this book. For those of you that are in the Central Florida area, I am offering you a consultation and examination to review your treatment options at my office for just $20. (Dental codes D0150 and D0274)

Please bring your copy of this book with you to your appointment to redeem this offer. Offer is good through December 31, 2020. You may share your book with multiple people; just have them bring it in with them for their initial consultations too.

Schroeder Dental Group

200 North Park Avenue

Suite A

Apopka Fl, 32703

(407) 886-1611

Implant Discussion Guide

On my website, www.ThePatientsGuidetoDentistry.com, you can request a discussion guide to take with you to your consultations.